The Mediterranean Diet for Every Day

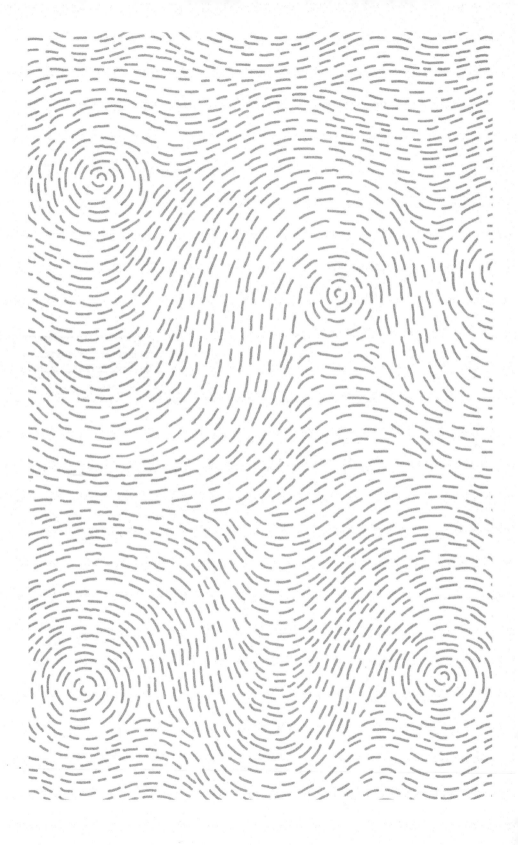

The Mediterranean Diet for Every Day

4 WEEKS OF RECIPES & MEAL PLANS
TO LOSE WEIGHT & IMPROVE HEALTH

TELAMON
PRESS

Contents

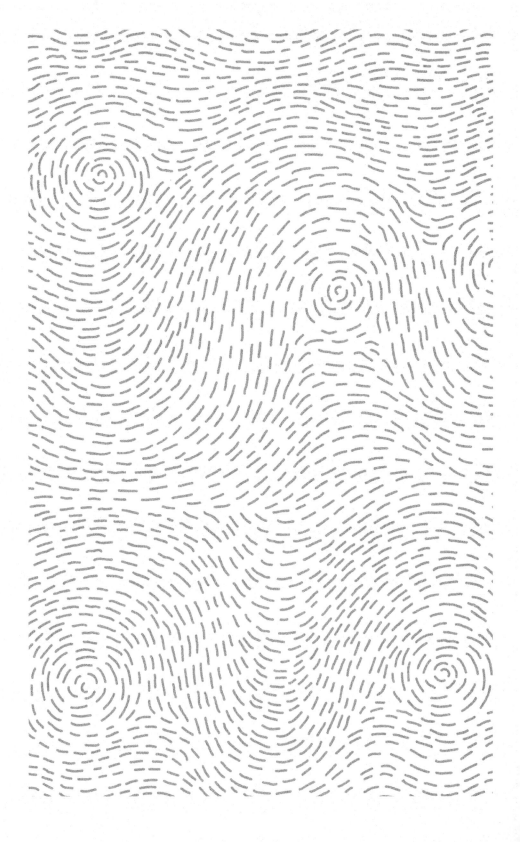

Introduction

When you hear the word "Mediterranean," what do you think of? Perhaps you envision crusty loaves of bread, tender olives, and fresh herbs. Or maybe you imagine a glass of red wine shared with friends. Better yet, you might picture yourself watching the sunset over a lush vineyard from the open deck of a grand Tuscan villa. All these things are characteristically "Mediterranean," but they do not define the Mediterranean lifestyle. In the same way, there is no single "Mediterranean diet" because the word "Mediterranean" is used to describe a group of more than fifteen different countries bordering the Mediterranean Sea.

You may be wondering what constitutes the Mediterranean diet trend that has recently become popular. Rather than prescribing a strict set of rules for foods to eat and foods to avoid, the Mediterranean diet offers guidelines for a healthful way of life. The Mediterranean diet is about more than just food, however—it is about living life to its fullest and being healthy as you do so. Life is meant to be shared and enjoyed, so you won't find restrictive calorie requirements or excessive exercise recommendations in this book. Here you will find a plan to transform your eating habits in a way that affects not only your health but also your entire life.

The Mediterranean diet is about eating wholesome foods such as fresh fruit and vegetables, bread, cereal grains, beans, nuts, and seeds. And who could forget olive oil, fresh fish, and good wine? In this book you will find more than one hundred delicious recipes that follow the principles of the Mediterranean diet, from hearty breakfasts and light lunches to satisfying dinners and delectable desserts. You will also learn in detail the benefits associated with the Mediterranean diet and the science behind it. With this book in your arsenal, you will be ready to transform your life by switching to the Mediterranean diet.

If you have ever tried a diet before, you may be worried about the difficulty of sticking to the Mediterranean diet. Your first step in making the switch is to leave those worries behind—this book will provide you with everything you need to get started on the right foot so you stick to the diet (and love every minute of it). You will receive background information on the diet itself, as well as shopping lists, cooking tips, and more. This book is arranged in an easy-to-understand fashion, leading you one day at a time through an entire four weeks of Mediterranean diet meals.

For many people, the most difficult part of sticking to a diet is finding recipes that are easy to prepare and full of flavor. With this book in hand, you definitely won't have that problem. Not only will you receive more than one hundred delicious recipes, but you will also receive a four-week meal plan to help you through your first month on the Mediterranean diet. After your first month you can choose to repeat the meal plan or to strike out on your own with the skills and tips you glean from this book. No matter which path you choose, you are sure to be amazed by the benefits you experience from following the Mediterranean diet. The Mediterranean diet has changed countless lives—what is stopping you from letting it change yours?

Getting Started

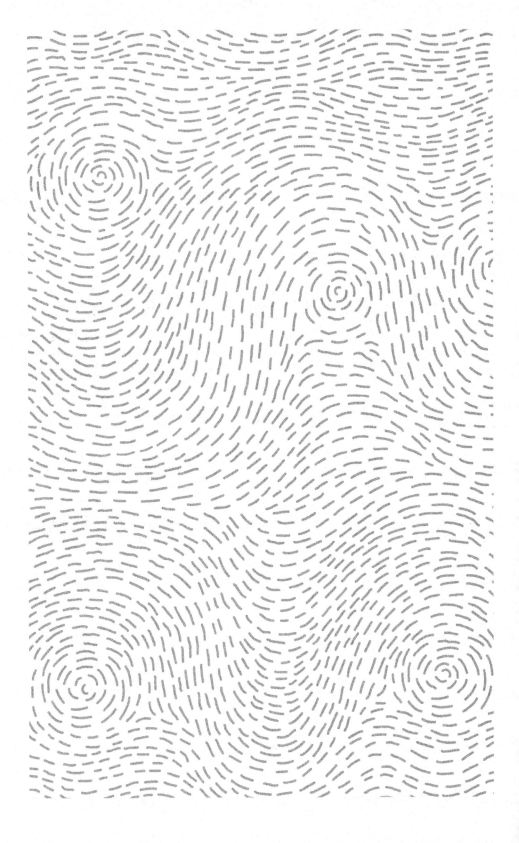

CHAPTER ONE

What Is the Mediterranean Diet?

Embracing the Mediterranean diet is all about making some simple but profound changes in the way you eat today, tomorrow, and for the rest of your life.

—Oldways Preservation Trust, "Mediterranean Diet 101"

As stated in the introduction, there is no one "Mediterranean diet." That is to say that all the countries bordering the Mediterranean Sea have their own unique cuisines and delicacies. Most Mediterranean cultures, however, follow similar dietary principles and habits, which is what the modern Mediterranean diet is based on. Before you can make the switch to the Mediterranean diet, you need to understand the basics: What are the benefits of this diet? Is it possible to lose weight on the Mediterranean diet? And which foods should be included and avoided on the diet?

There are many different diet plans available to choose from, and you might be overwhelmed by the sheer number of choices. The Mediterranean diet is just one of those choices, but you will soon see why it is superior to many other options. In this chapter you will learn everything you need to know in order to make an educated decision regarding whether the Mediterranean diet is the right choice for you. If it is, you can move on to the second chapter of this book, in which you will learn how to effectively utilize the tools and meal plans included in this book. Your journey in weight loss and health transformation begins here, so don't be afraid to jump right in.

BENEFITS OF THE DIET

In 2012, the American Heart Association (AHA) published an assessment of the Mediterranean diet and how well it adheres to the AHA's standards for heart-healthy eating. The AHA found that the average Mediterranean diet is lower in saturated fat than the traditional American diet—in fact, the average consumption rate of saturated fat in Mediterranean cultures is well within the AHA dietary guidelines. Though the Mediterranean diet is high in dietary fat, more than half of the fat calories consumed in the Mediterranean diet come from monounsaturated fat. Monounsaturated fat, which comes from sources like olive oil and avocados, has a lesser effect on blood cholesterol levels than saturated fat, which comes from animal products such as meat, eggs, and dairy. The AHA also found that death rates and the incidence of heart disease were lower in Mediterranean countries, although the more active lifestyle of many Mediterranean cultures compared with the average American activity level is considered to be a significant factor in this statistic.

Though improved heart health and reduced risk for heart disease are two of the main benefits of the Mediterranean diet, they are not the only benefits. In the years following World War II, Dr. Ancel Keys, a Minnesota physiologist, helped pilot a study on the effects of the Mediterranean diet on overall health. This study involved more than twelve thousand middle-aged men from seven different countries, thus earning it the name the Seven Countries Study (Keys, 1966). The countries represented in this study include the United States, Italy, Japan, Greece, Finland, Yugoslavia, and the Netherlands. The study began in 1958, and the results were published in book form by Harvard University Press in 1980. The main focus of the study was to determine the preventability of heart disease and the effects of saturated fat consumption on heart health, but the results were just the tip of the iceberg in scientific research regarding the Mediterranean diet (Keys, 1966).

Following the findings of the Seven Countries Study, many other studies were conducted regarding the various health benefits of the Mediterranean diet. A study published in the *British Medical Journal* in 2008, for example, revealed that adherence to a Mediterranean diet was associated with a 9 percent reduction in overall mortality in test subjects as well as a 13 percent reduction in risk for neurodegenerative diseases such as Alzheimer's and Parkinson's disease (Sofi et al., 2008). In 2009, a study was published in the *Journal of Nutrition* regarding the effect of the Mediterranean diet on the risk for chronic disease. The results of this study suggest that an eating pattern high in plant foods and unsaturated fats, like the Mediterranean diet, can reduce the risk for lower abdominal obesity and coronary heart disease (Romaguera et al., 2009).

Combined with regular exercise and not smoking, the Mediterranean diet can greatly reduce your risk for chronic disease. A study published in the *Journal of Public Health and Nutrition* in 2006 revealed that these healthful choices can help prevent over 70 percent of strokes, 90 percent of cases of type 2 diabetes, and 80 percent of instances of coronary heart disease (Romaguera et al., 2006).

In addition to preventing heart disease, the Mediterranean diet has been linked in several studies to reduced risk for certain cancers. A study published in the *American Journal of Epidemiology* followed the eating habits of more than sixty-five thousand women and revealed that following the Mediterranean diet can reduce the risk for postmenopausal breast cancer (Cottet et al. 2009). A review of more than twenty thousand cases published in 2009 further revealed that increased consumption of fruits, vegetables, whole grains, and fish reduced the risk for epithelial cancer cell growth. The same review showed that monounsaturated fat consumption was inversely related to cancer risk at more than twenty different cancer sites (La Vecchia, 2009).

The results of a Spanish study suggest that olive oil consumption could help protect women against breast cancer. Consumption of as little as ten teaspoons a day of olive oil could significantly reduce your risk for cancer. The study revealed that olive oil helps attack cancer cells from multiple angles by stunting tumor growth and preventing cancerous damage to the DNA of cells (*Science Daily*, 2006).

As is true of any diet, the health benefits associated with the Mediterranean diet can vary from one individual to another. Some of the other benefits followers of the Mediterranean diet have reported include reduced risk for diabetes, relief from rheumatoid arthritis, improved eye health, improved fertility, relief from depression and other mood disorders, improved brain function, and increased longevity. Following the Mediterranean diet can also help you lose weight and maintain a healthful body mass index (BMI). You will learn more about this in the next section.

LOSING WEIGHT ON THE MEDITERRANEAN DIET

It is possible to lose weight with nearly any diet as long as you follow the guidelines and burn more calories than you consume. The problem with many diets, however, is that the guidelines themselves are very strict or confusing, which makes it hard to stick to them. The Mediterranean diet, however, is a fairly easy concept to understand, and as long as you engage in healthful eating habits, you should have no trouble losing weight. In fact, several recent studies have shown that losing weight on the Mediterranean diet is a very likely outcome.

A study published in the *Journal of Nutrition* in 2008 studied the effect of Mediterranean-style eating patterns on the modification of food habits. The results of the study showed that the Mediterranean diet not only helps modify eating habits, but can also reduce the over-caloric density of one's diet (Goulet, Lamarche, and Lemieux, 2008). Other studies have shown that the Mediterranean diet can be an excellent alternative to a low-fat, high-carb diet. Though the average Mediterranean diet includes 20 percent or more calories from fat, those calories are derived from heart-healthy monounsaturated fats, not the saturated fats that are thought to contribute to obesity.

· ·

Try using heart-healthy oils as a replacement for butter in cooking. Drizzle a teaspoon of olive oil over steamed vegetables or toss them in a dab of coconut oil. Try some flavored oils, like garlic -or rosemary-infused olive oil, to give bread and vegetables additional flavor without the added fat.

· ·

Now that you know a little bit about the Mediterranean diet and its potential to help you lose weight, you may be wondering just how it works. As has already been mentioned, you can lose weight on almost any diet, so what makes the Mediterranean diet different? One component of the Mediterranean diet involves eating more fruits and vegetables. Fruits and vegetables are nutrient-dense foods, which means they have a high proportion of nutrients to calories; these foods are much lower in calories than many processed snack foods. Whole grains, another component of the Mediterranean diet, are also richer in nutrients than refined and processed grains like white rice, bleached flour, and processed bread. By eating more nutrient-rich foods like these, which are also high in fiber, you will feel fuller longer on fewer calories.

The Mediterranean diet also helps you lose weight by encouraging healthful food swaps—that is, substituting healthier options for high-fat and high-calorie foods. For example, the traditional American diet often incorporates butter as a cooking fat. In the Mediterranean diet, however, olive oil and canola oil are recommended; these options are a good source of mono-unsaturated, as opposed to saturated, fats. The type of protein you eat when following the Mediterranean diet will also play a role in helping you achieve your weight-loss goals. While many diets are based on fried foods and red meat, the Mediterranean diet focuses on lean protein sources such as fish and poultry, limiting red meat to a few portions per month.

The dangers of eating too much red meat may not be limited to saturated fat content. A recent study revealed that L-carnitine, a nutrient found in red meat, can interact with certain bacteria in the gut. This interaction might cause cholesterol removal to slow, thus clogging arteries and increasing the risk for heart problems (Lopatto, 2013).

The key to losing weight while following the Mediterranean diet is to make healthful eating choices. Many of the foods included in the diet are naturally lower in calories or fat than many of the foods that make up the staples of the modern Western diet. Of course you do still need to be mindful of how much you are eating. The Mediterranean diet does not prescribe specific calorie counts, but you should pay attention to proper portion sizes and make an effort not to overeat. Drinking plenty of water and rounding out your meals with low-calorie side dishes like salads and steamed vegetables will help fill you up while keeping your daily calorie count down. Later in this book, you will receive additional tips for losing weight while following the Mediterranean diet.

FOODS TO INCLUDE AND AVOID

Now that you understand the basics of the Mediterranean diet, you may be ready to get into the details—what can you eat? Because the Mediterranean diet is all about healthful eating habits and enjoying the food you eat, you should try not to think of these guidelines in terms of what you cannot eat. Too many diets place heavy restrictions on the foods you can eat, which leave people feeling dissatisfied. The foods included in the Mediterranean diet are full of natural flavor, and there are many ways to dress up your meals, so you should never feel deprived.

The main foods included in the Mediterranean diet are as follows:

- Extra-virgin olive oil
- Fresh fish and seafood
- Fresh, frozen, and canned fruits
- Fresh, frozen, and canned vegetables
- Fresh herbs and spices
- Nonfat Greek yogurt
- Nuts and seeds
- Olives and avocados
- Part-skim milk cheese
- Potatoes and legumes
- Poultry (chicken, turkey, etc.)
- Skim milk
- Whole-grain bread and pasta
- Whole grains (brown rice, cereal grains, etc.)

Foods to limit on the Mediterranean diet include:

- High-fat dairy products (whole or 2 percent milk, ice cream, etc.)
- Natural sweeteners (raw sugar, honey, maple syrup, stevia, etc.)
- Red meat (three to four servings per month)
- Wine (one glass per day with meals)

Foods you should avoid when possible are as follows:

- Fatty cuts of meat
- Fried foods and fast food
- Processed snacks and prepared foods

- Refined sugar and flour
- Saturated fats (butter, margarine, etc.)
- Sugary desserts and candy

LOOKING AHEAD

In this chapter you learned the basics of the Mediterranean diet, including its origins, the associated health benefits, and its potential to help you meet your weight-loss goals. You also received an overview of the foods that should be included, limited, and avoided while following the diet. In the next chapter you will receive information and actionable steps regarding forming and following your Mediterranean diet meal plan. You will also receive a collection of cooking tips and steps for success in switching to the Mediterranean diet.

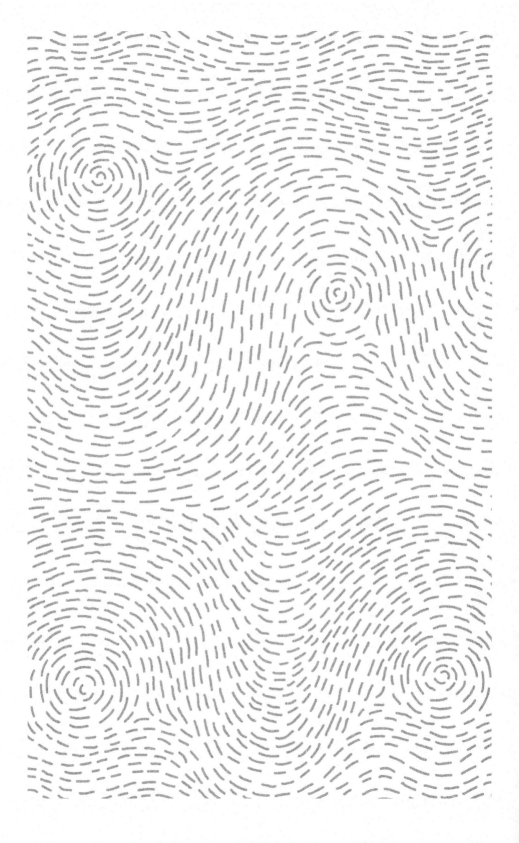

CHAPTER TWO

How to Use the Meal Plan

You can have a big impact on your health—and your budget— just by eating at home more often. With menu planning you know what your meals will look like and what you need to buy ... Menu planning doesn't have to be complicated!

—Mayo Clinic Staff, "Menu Planning: Eat Healthier and Spend Less"

Many people struggle to stick to their new diets for more than a week because of one simple reason: boredom. If you feel as if you are stuck eating the same things day in and day out, you are more likely to succumb to your cravings and step outside the guidelines of the diet. Once you do that, it is only a matter of time before you abandon the diet entirely. Creating a meal plan for each week is a simple and effective way to keep yourself on track with the Mediterranean diet. By having a meal plan in front of you, you can be assured that each meal you enjoy is unique. You also have the convenience of doing all your shopping ahead of time so as not to have to make any last-minute decisions. Additionally, having a meal plan will help you use your groceries more efficiently to cut down on waste, which will also save some of your hard-earned money.

CREATING AND IMPLEMENTING A MEAL PLAN

Creating a weekly meal plan for the Mediterranean diet is easy—especially when you already have more than one hundred delicious recipes to incorporate. A meal plan is nothing more than a list of meals you intend to prepare in the coming week, so all you have to do is choose what you want to eat.

Follow the tips below to create and implement your weekly meal plan:

1. Go through your recipes and make a pile or list of things you'd like to try. Include some for each course (including dessert).
2. Separate the recipes into piles for each course: breakfast, lunch, dinner, and dessert.
3. On a pad of paper (or on your computer) make a heading for Day One through Day Seven with enough space below each to list four meals.
4. Start with your pile of breakfast recipes and choose one for each day, writing it below the proper heading.

Expedite your meal planning using a computer-based spreadsheet program. If you are skilled with a computer, you will be able to design an interactive spreadsheet that allows you to create new plans by scrambling the recipes you have already input. For basic users, however, it is still easy to list your recipes in a spreadsheet so you can copy and paste the names under the appropriate days. This is also a great method if you want to repeat an entire day's or week's worth of meals.

5. Repeat this process with lunch, dinner, and dessert until your meal plan is complete.
6. Glance through the individual recipes, making a list of the pantry items and groceries you will need to get through the week.
7. Do the necessary shopping the day before you intend to implement your meal plan. You can shop once for the week or divide it into two trips if you prefer.
8. Store the purchased foods so they will last the week. If you buy a roast for Day Six, for example, be sure it will last that long, or freeze it until the evening of Day Five so it is fresh.
9. Follow your meal plan. Simply prepare the recipes you've chosen on the assigned days (it is as easy as that).

MAKING A GROCERY LIST

When making a grocery list to use in conjunction with your meal plan, there are a few things you can do to make the process simpler. As you are going through your recipes for the week, take note of not only the items you need but also the quantity. For example, if you are making Spiced Sweet Potato Pancakes, you should write down that you will need two eggs, one cup skim milk, one cup baking mix, etc. You may find it easier to make a bulleted list of basic items (milk, eggs, flour, etc.) and simply put a tally next to the item to denote a certain quantity (one cup, one egg, etc.). At the end, you can total your tallies and figure out how much of each item on your list you actually need.

A sample grocery list might look something like this:

Mediterranean Diet
MEAL PLAN WEEK ONE

Pantry Items:

All-purpose flour (3 cups)

Baking mix (2 cups)

Extra-virgin olive oil

Sea salt

Dried oregano

Dried basil

Meat and Protein:

Eggs – (whole) IIIII IIII

Boneless chicken breast –
    (whole) III

Raw shrimp – 1½ lbs.

Ground turkey – 1 lb.

Boneless halibut fillets – (4 oz.) IIII

Fresh Produce:

Bananas - (whole) IIII

Lemons– (whole) II

Fresh basil – 1 bunch

Fresh parsley – 2 bunches

Kale – 2 bunches

Yellow onions – (whole) III

Plum tomatoes – (small) IIII

Carrots – 1 bag

Celery – 1 bag

Sweet potatoes (whole) III

Dairy:

Skim milk – (cups) IIII

Heavy cream (cups) I

Other Items:

Whole-wheat pasta – 1 box

Diced tomatoes – 2 large cans

Whole garlic – 1 head

Whole-grain bread – 1 loaf

Raisins – (cups) I

LEARNING TO READ FOOD LABELS

Reading food labels at the grocery store can be tricky, especially when marketing companies word things in a way that can skew your perception. Take a quick walk down the snack aisle at your local grocery store. What jumps out at you? Perhaps colorful, bold fonts draw your eye, or maybe you are sucked in by "low-fat," "sugar-free," or "reduced-fat" claims. These are just a few of the tactics marketing companies and food manufacturers use to entice customers to buy their products. While the claims may be based in fact, things are not always as simple and straightforward as they seem.

Take a look at the nutrition facts for a loaf of sandwich bread. You will see the serving size listed at the top along with the calories per serving, calories from fat, and the content per serving of various nutrients, including fat, cholesterol, sodium, carbohydrates, dietary fiber, sugar, and protein. You will also find an ingredients list that will tell you, in order of weight, the ingredients used to create the product. Here you would expect to find ingredients like eggs, flour, and milk. You may, however, find some ingredients you were not expecting and others that you do not understand.

Beware of food products that contain sugar alcohols. In an effort to label a product "sugar-free," many manufacturers have turned to using sugar alcohols instead of natural sugar. Keep in mind that these ingredients are not necessarily calorie-free and they often cause gastrointestinal stress. To identify sugar alcohols, look for names like sorbitol, xylitol, and mannitol.

It is important to keep in mind that the order in which the ingredients are listed is just as important as the ingredients themselves. Ingredients listed near the beginning are present in higher quantities than ingredients listed farther down. Many food manufacturers sneak in extra sugar and preservatives to make their products taste better and last longer, but these ingredients are not good for your health. Even if a product is listed as "all-natural," it could still contain a lot of corn syrup or salt.

When examining food labels at the grocery store, you should look for products with short ingredient lists (fewer ingredients means fewer unnatural additives) and whole ingredients. Whole-grain flour, for example, is better for you than enriched flour. It may take some getting used to, but if you take the time to look at the labels on the food you are purchasing, it might help you make healthier choices. At the very least, it might help you move past the sugary cereals and snacks and on to healthier items.

MEDITERRANEAN COOKING TIPS

If you are not used to cooking for yourself or your family, it may take you some time to get used to following a recipe. Here is a list of definitions for common cooking methods you'll use when following the recipes that are included in this book:

- **Al dente:** a term used to describe pasta that has been cooked to the ideal level—it should be tender with a slight resistance to the bite
- **Beat:** to mix quickly; often done using an electric hand mixer
- **Broil:** to cook under strong, direct heat
- **Brown:** to cook an item (usually meat) quickly over high heat so the outside turns brown
- **Chop:** to cut into solid pieces, generally less than one inch
- **Dice:** to cut into small pieces, generally half an inch or less
- **Dredge:** to coat or sprinkle an item with flour before cooking
- **Fold:** to incorporate a light or delicate substance into a mixture without releasing air bubbles; commonly used for whipped cream, beaten eggs, etc.
- **Marinate:** to soak an item in a liquid mixture before cooking to impart flavor; may be brushed on during cooking as well
- **Mince:** to chop an item into extremely small pieces, e.g., garlic
- **Purée:** to mash foods until smooth by hand, in a blender, or in a food processor
- **Sauté:** to cook and/or brown a food in hot fat or oil
- **Simmer:** to cook slowly in liquid over low heat

In addition to these tips, you may find it helpful to know what kind of equipment you'll need. The staple items you will be called on to use include skillets and saucepans of varying size. You might also need an electric griddle (a heavy nonstick skillet will work as well), a blender, a food processor, a mixer, and an assortment of glass and metal baking dishes. If you are not used to cooking, simply follow the instructions in the recipes as closely as possible. Over time you will get the hang of certain cooking methods and you will no longer find it difficult at all.

TEN STEPS FOR SUCCESS

Follow these easy tips for success when you start out on the Mediterranean diet:

1. Have a collection of healthful snacks on hand for those moments when hunger strikes. Try carrots and hummus, apple chips, or a healthful salad.
2. Incorporate vegetables and fruits into your diet in fun ways. Try baked kale chips, sweet potato fries, or zucchini muffins.
3. Keep plenty of Mediterranean diet staples on hand. Your pantry should be stocked with whole-grain flours, extra-virgin olive oil, diced tomatoes, olives, and plenty of dried spices.
4. Incorporate fruit into your daily routine in snacks and at breakfast. Have half a banana with your morning meal or eat an apple when you take a break at work.
5. Make meals fun! It isn't a rule that diets have to be boring. Make cooking a family affair and enjoy your mealtime together.
6. Don't be afraid to have that glass of wine. Drinking wine with dinner is actually encouraged in the Mediterranean diet.
7. Experiment with new flavors. Top your salads with feta cheese or chopped olives, add roasted red peppers to your morning eggs, or make a smoothie using leftovers from last night's salad.
8. Eat plenty of lean protein. You should be eating seafood at least twice a week on the Mediterranean diet and limiting red meat to three or four portions per month.
9. Visit your local farmers, market for fresh produce and great cooking ideas. Everything tastes better—and is often more nutritious—when it's fresh.
10. Mix things up. Once you finish the four weeks of meal plans in this book, use the included recipes (as well as some of your own) to create new meal plans.

Following the Mediterranean diet should be fun, not a chore. By following these simple steps and incorporating the tips you learned earlier in the chapter, you should have no trouble sticking to the diet.

LOOKING AHEAD

In this chapter you learned the basics about what meal planning is and how it can benefit you and your family while you're following the Mediterranean diet. Meal planning not only is a convenient way to organize your weekly meals, but it can also save you time and money. You also learned how to make an efficient grocery list and how to read food labels at the grocery store, and you received some helpful tips for success. In the next section of this book you will receive four week-long meal plans, plus the recipes for all of the breakfasts, lunches, dinners, and desserts listed in the meal plans so you can get started with the Mediterranean diet.

Now that you understand the basics of the Mediterranean diet and have been educated on the benefits of using a meal plan, you are ready to start one yourself. As was mentioned in the last chapter, all that you have to do in order to implement the meal plans in this book is to follow the grocery lists and prepare the listed meals on the appropriate days. It is recommended that you follow the first week of the meal plan completely in order to get used to the guidelines of the Mediterranean diet, and to get yourself into some healthful eating habits. After the first week, however, you can swap a few recipes from the book here and there according to your preferences.

Part Two of this book is broken into four sections, one for each week. Each week includes a seven-day meal plan with four meals per day—breakfast, lunch, dinner, and dessert—as well as a recipe for each meal. Snacks are also listed, though recipes for the snacks are not provided; you will find more information about these snacks in the appendices at the end of the book. Familiarize yourself with the week's meal plan, then go over the shopping list to see what you need to purchase. Remember, you may already have some of the pantry items in stock. Once you have done your shopping, view and follow the Plan-Ahead Preparations for the week. All that is left then is to get started. Every day in the meal plan has a relevant tip to help you with your journey in following the Mediterranean diet. You will also find a section of additional tips at the end of each week.

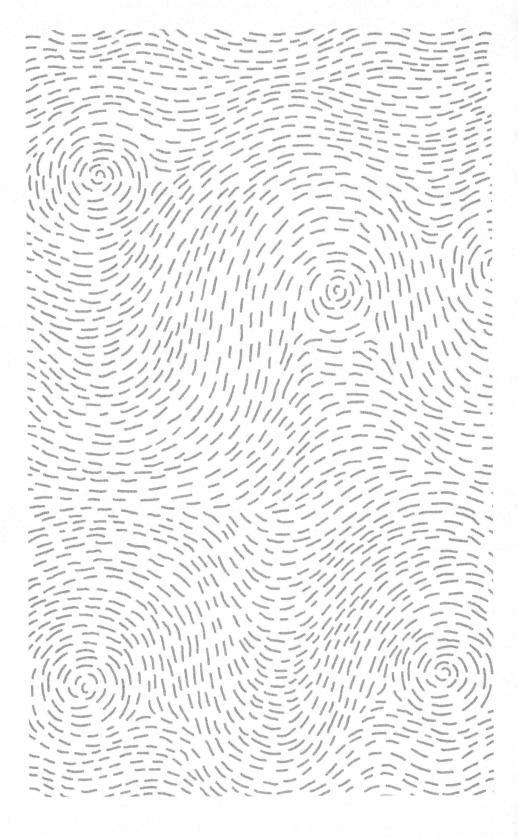

PART TWO

Putting the Meal Plan into Action

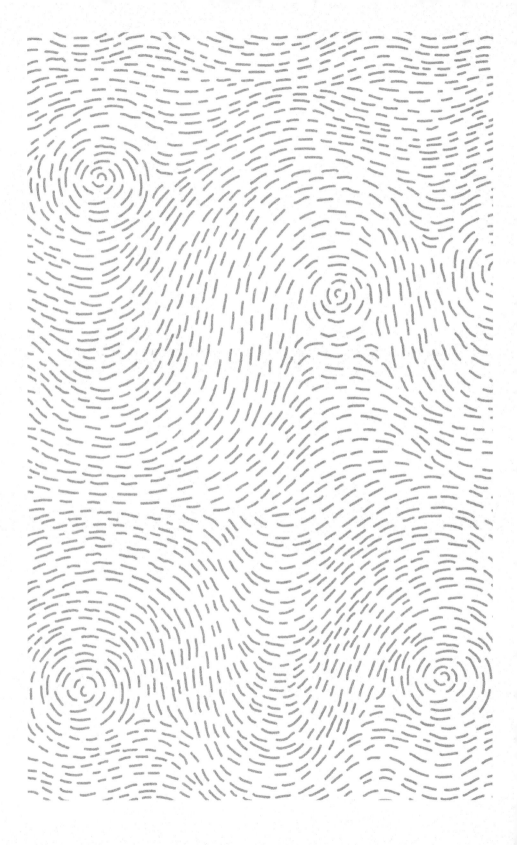

CHAPTER THREE

Week One

The Mediterranean Diet isn't just one more fad to follow. It's a healthy way of eating that can help everyone live a longer life and lower the risk of disease. It also offers many nutritious ways to help [you] improve [your] lifelong health.

—Oldways Preservation Trust, "Tips for Women"

WEEK ONE MEAL PLAN

Day One

Breakfast: Cinnamon Apple Breakfast Couscous
Lunch: Tuna Salad with Capers and Olives
Dinner: Italian-Herbed Lamb Chops
Snacks: 2 tablespoons hummus with 8 baby carrots; 1 small sliced apple
Dessert: Simple Lemon Sorbet

Daily Tip: To boost your weight-loss efforts, try to incorporate thirty minutes of moderate exercise three times per week. This can be as simple as a walk through the park on your lunch break or taking your dog for a jog after work.

Day Two

Breakfast: Pineapple Kale Smoothie
Lunch: Three-Bean Greek Salad
Dinner: Mediterranean Chicken Stew
Snacks: 4 whole-grain crackers; 1 sliced tomato with 1 tablespoon grated Parmesan cheese
Dessert: Chocolate-Covered Figs

> **Daily Tip:** Try to slow down during your meals. If you eat too quickly, you may end up with a false sense of hunger after you have already completed the meal.

Day Three

Breakfast: Tomato Basil Omelet
Lunch: Shaved Lamb Lettuce Wraps
Dinner: Goat Cheese–Stuffed Tomatoes
Snacks: 2 tablespoons toasted chickpeas; ½ cup plain nonfat Greek yogurt mixed with 1 teaspoon honey
Dessert: Spiced Rice Pudding

> **Daily Tip:** Don't be overly concerned with counting calories, but make an effort to keep your portion sizes appropriate. Follow the serving size guidelines on the package when possible.

Day Four

Breakfast: Banana Walnut Bread
Lunch: Grilled Vegetable Skewers
Dinner: Maple Lime Salmon
Snacks: 3 tablespoons dried fruit; 15 whole almonds
Dessert: Peanut Butter Oatmeal Balls

Daily Tip: Remember that you do not have to be perfect in order to reach your goals. Success in following the Mediterranean diet is a marathon and not a sprint, so don't get too down on yourself if you make a little mistake.

Day Five

Breakfast: Baked Eggs with Goat Cheese
Lunch: Cream of Avocado Soup
Dinner: Broiled Turkey Burgers with Arugula
Snacks: 1 tablespoon hummus with celery; 4 whole-grain crackers
Dessert: Strawberry Almond Smoothie

Daily Tip: Make an effort to drink plenty of water during the day. Drink at least eight ounces of water an hour before exercise and with every meal to stay hydrated.

Day Six

Breakfast: Spiced Sweet Potato Pancakes
Lunch: Chopped Beet and Arugula Salad
Dinner: Winter Vegetable Ragout
Snacks: 1 small baked apple with cinnamon; 1 peach
Dessert: Honey-Glazed Almonds

Daily Tip: Incorporate activity into your daily routine in fun or unique ways. Take the stairs instead of the elevator, race your kids from the car into the house, or simply make an effort to keep moving throughout the day.

Day Seven

Breakfast: Blueberry Almond Granola
Lunch: Butternut Squash Soup
Dinner: Lemon-Basil Shrimp and Linguine
Snacks: Toasted pumpkin seeds; pitted olives
Dessert: Cinnamon-Walnut Biscotti

. . . .

Daily Tip: Take the time to enjoy a family meal. If you eat at the dinner table with family (instead of in front of the TV), you will be more focused on the meal and are likely to feel more satisfied afterward than you would after mindless eating.

. . . .

Note: The snacks included in this meal plan are simple snacks you can purchase from the grocery store that need little to no preparation. For more information regarding the nutritional content of these snacks, refer to Appendix A.

ADDITIONAL TIPS FOR WEEK ONE:

- Don't be afraid to use leftovers. Slice up the lamb from dinner on Day One to use in your lettuce wraps on Day Three.
- Be patient with yourself. If you are used to following a diet of fast food or frozen dinners, it will take time to get used to cooking for yourself.
- Give yourself plenty of time in the grocery store. If you don't normally spend much time shopping, you should take the time to learn where things are (it will make future trips much quicker).
- Don't feel as if you have to buy what is available. Sometimes you can find produce of a much higher quality at your local food co-op or farmers, market than you can at your big-name grocery store.
- View each day on the Mediterranean diet as an opportunity to try something new and to improve your health.

WEEK ONE RECIPES

Breakfast Recipes

CINNAMON APRICOT BREAKFAST COUSCOUS

PINEAPPLE KALE SMOOTHIE

TOMATO BASIL OMELET

BANANA WALNUT BREAD

BAKED EGGS WITH GOAT CHEESE

SPICED SWEET POTATO PANCAKES

BLUEBERRY ALMOND GRANOLA

Lunch Recipes

TUNA SALAD WITH CAPERS AND OLIVES

THREE-BEAN GREEK SALAD

SHAVED LAMB LETTUCE WRAPS

GRILLED VEGETABLE SKEWERS

CREAM OF AVOCADO SOUP

CHOPPED BEET AND ARUGULA SALAD

BUTTERNUT SQUASH SOUP

Dinner Recipes

ITALIAN-HERBED LAMB CHOPS

MEDITERRANEAN CHICKEN STEW

GOAT CHEESE-STUFFED TOMATOES

MAPLE LIME SALMON

BROILED TURKEY BURGERS WITH ARUGULA

WINTER VEGETABLE RAGOUT

LEMON-BASIL SHRIMP AND LINGUINE

Dessert Recipes

SIMPLE LEMON SORBET

CHOCOLATE-COVERED FIGS

SPICED RICE PUDDING

PEANUT BUTTER OATMEAL BALLS

STRAWBERRY ALMOND SMOOTHIE

HONEY-GLAZED ALMONDS

CINNAMON-WALNUT BISCOTTI

Breakfast Recipes

Cinnamon Apricot Breakfast Couscous

SERVES 4

You may be used to seeing couscous as a side dish for a main meal, but this recipe will show you just how delicious it can be for breakfast. Simply sweeten it with brown sugar and flavor it with cinnamon for a delightfully easy morning meal.

3 CUPS SKIM MILK

ONE 2-INCH CINNAMON STICK

1 CUP DRY WHOLE-WHEAT COUSCOUS

½ CUP DRIED APRICOTS, CHOPPED

¼ CUP RAISINS

5 TEASPOONS BROWN SUGAR

PINCH OF SALT

4 TEASPOONS CANOLA OIL

1. Pour the milk into a medium saucepan and drop in the cinnamon stick. Heat the milk over medium-high heat until small bubbles form around the edges.

2. Remove the saucepan from heat and stir in the remaining ingredients, reserving 1 teaspoon of brown sugar.

3. Cover and let the couscous stand for 10 to 15 minutes, or until the couscous absorbs the liquid. Remove and discard the cinnamon stick.

4. Sprinkle the remaining teaspoon of brown sugar on top to serve.

Pineapple Kale Smoothie

SERVES 2

Smoothies are a quick and simple way to start your day. This smoothie is the perfect combination of sweet pineapple flavor and nutritious kale.

2 CUPS FROZEN CHOPPED PINEAPPLE

1 CUP CHOPPED KALE

1 CUP ORANGE JUICE

½ CUP PLAIN NONFAT GREEK YOGURT

1 TEASPOON HONEY (OPTIONAL)

½ CUP ICE CUBES

1. Place the pineapple, kale, and orange juice in a blender and blend for 30 seconds on high speed.

2. Add the yogurt, honey (if using), and ice and blend until smooth.

3. Pour the smoothie into two glasses and serve immediately.

Tomato Basil Omelet

SERVES 1

This omelet utilizes fresh ingredients to make a meal that will satisfy your hunger and keep you feeling full throughout the morning.

2 EGGS

1 TABLESPOON SKIM MILK

½ TEASPOON SALT

¼ TEASPOON FRESHLY GROUND PEPPER

2 TEASPOONS EXTRA-VIRGIN OLIVE OIL

1 MEDIUM PLUM TOMATO, CHOPPED

1 SMALL SHALLOT, MINCED

¼ CUP CHOPPED FRESH BASIL

1. Crack the eggs into a small bowl and whisk in the skim milk, salt, and pepper until well combined. Set the bowl aside.

2. Heat 1 teaspoon of olive oil in a small skillet over medium heat.

3. Stir in the tomato, shallot, and basil and cook for 2 to 3 minutes, or until hot.

4. Spoon the tomato mixture into a bowl and set aside.

5. Heat the remaining teaspoon of olive oil in the same skillet and pour in the egg mixture. Rotate the pan to coat the sides with egg.

6. Let the eggs cook for 1 minute; then scrape down the sides of the pan using a spatula, letting the uncooked eggs spread.

7. Allow the eggs to cook for 1 to 2 minutes longer, or until almost set. Spoon the tomato mixture over half of the omelet.

8. Fold the empty half of the omelet over the tomato filling and allow the eggs to cook for 1 more minute, or until the eggs are cooked through. Serve hot.

Banana Walnut Bread

MAKES 1 LOAF

Banana bread is a staple, well loved for breakfast and snacks alike. This recipe adheres well to the Mediterranean diet principles because it utilizes whole-wheat flour, skim milk, and chopped nuts.

COOKING SPRAY

2 CUPS MASHED BANANA

½ CUP CANOLA OIL

2 EGGS

1 CUP SUGAR

¼ CUP SKIM MILK

¾ TEASPOON VANILLA EXTRACT

1 CUP WHOLE-WHEAT FLOUR

1 CUP UNBLEACHED FLOUR

1 TEASPOON BAKING SODA

½ TEASPOON BAKING POWDER

½ TEASPOON SALT

2 TEASPOONS GROUND CINNAMON

PINCH OF GROUND NUTMEG

⅔ CUP CHOPPED WALNUTS

1. Preheat the oven to 350°F.

2. Lightly grease a regular loaf pan with cooking spray.

3. Whisk together the mashed banana, canola oil, eggs, sugar, milk, and vanilla extract in a large mixing bowl.

4. In a separate bowl, stir together the flours, baking soda, baking powder, salt, cinnamon, and nutmeg.

5. Stir the dry ingredients into the wet until the mixture is well combined. Fold in the chopped walnuts.

6. Spoon the batter into the prepared pan and bake for 60 to 75 minutes, or until a knife inserted in the center of the loaf comes out clean.

7. Remove the loaf from the oven and let it stand for 10 minutes.

8. Turn the loaf out onto a wire rack to cool completely before cutting.

Baked Eggs with Goat Cheese

SERVES 4

These baked eggs are surprisingly easy to make but will certainly impress your family. Flavored with freshly ground pepper, and supplemented with tender spinach and goat cheese, eggs have never tasted this good.

COOKING SPRAY

3 TO 4 TABLESPOONS PLAIN BREAD CRUMBS

3 TABLESPOONS EXTRA-VIRGIN OLIVE OIL

¼ CUP FINELY CHOPPED ONION

1 TEASPOON FRESHLY GROUND PEPPER

½ TEASPOON SALT

4 CUPS CHOPPED SPINACH

1 TABLESPOON WATER

1 CUP CHOPPED TOMATOES

4 EGGS

½ CUP GOAT CHEESE CRUMBLES

1. Preheat the oven to 400°F.

2. Grease four 6- to 8-ounce ceramic ramekins with cooking spray.

3. Spoon up to 1 tablespoon of bread crumbs into the bottom of each ramekin and place them on a baking sheet.

4. Pour the olive oil into a large skillet and heat it over medium heat.

5. Stir in the onion, pepper, and salt. Cook for 2 to 3 minutes, or until the onions are just tender.

6. Stir in the chopped spinach and water and cook for 4 to 6 minutes, or until the spinach is tender and the water has evaporated.

7. Carefully spoon about ¼ cup of the spinach and onion mixture into each ramekin.

8. Top the spinach mixture with the chopped tomatoes, dividing them evenly among the four ramekins.

9. Use a spoon to make a hollow depression in the center of each ramekin. Crack an egg into the middle of each ramekin in the depression.

10. Sprinkle the goat cheese over the eggs and bake for 16 to 18 minutes, or until the egg whites are just set.

11. Let stand for 10 minutes before serving.

Spiced Sweet Potato Pancakes

SERVES 6

*If you are a fan of pancakes, these sweet and spicy pancakes are sure to satisfy.
The subtle sweetness of the sweet potato is perfectly offset by a hint of ground
nutmeg and cinnamon.*

2 EGGS

1 CUP SKIM MILK

2½ TABLESPOONS CANOLA OIL

1 CUP BAKING MIX

PINCH OF GROUND NUTMEG

PINCH OF GROUND CINNAMON

1½ CUPS BOILED, MASHED SWEET POTATO

1. Whisk together the eggs, milk, and canola oil in a mixing bowl.

2. In another bowl, stir together the baking mix, nutmeg, and cinnamon.
Add the dry mixture to the wet and whisk until smooth.

3. Fold in the sweet potato and set aside.

4. Heat a nonstick skillet over medium-high heat. Spoon the batter onto the
hot skillet in heaping tablespoons.

5. Let the pancakes cook until the batter begins to bubble on the surface,
1 to 2 minutes. Carefully flip the pancakes and cook for 1 to 2 minutes more, or
until the underside is lightly browned.

6. Transfer the cooked pancakes to a plate cover them to keep them warm.
Repeat until all the batter is used. Serve the pancakes warm with fresh fruit.

Blueberry Almond Granola

SERVES 6

Granola makes a wonderful breakfast food because it can be quite filling. Made with whole grains and flavored with dried blueberries and almonds, this recipe is sure to become a breakfast favorite.

2 CUPS OLD-FASHIONED OATS

⅓ CUP SLIVERED ALMONDS

¼ CUP CHOPPED WALNUTS

1 TEASPOON GROUND CINNAMON

PINCH OF SALT

3 TABLESPOONS CANOLA OIL

¼ CUP HONEY

¼ CUP PACKED BROWN SUGAR

1 TEASPOON ALMOND EXTRACT

½ CUP DRIED BLUEBERRIES

1. Preheat the oven to 375°F.

2. Line a rimmed baking sheet with parchment paper.

3. Combine the old-fashioned oats, almonds, and walnuts in a large mixing bowl with the cinnamon and salt. Toss well.

4. In a small bowl, whisk together the canola oil, honey, brown sugar, and almond extract.

5. Pour the canola oil mixture over the oat mixture and mix well by hand until the oats are coated. Spread the oat mixture out on the prepared baking sheet.

6. Bake for 10 minutes, then turn the granola with a spatula and bake 5 to 10 minutes more, or until just browned.

7. Transfer the mixture to a large bowl to cool and toss in the dried blueberries. Store in an airtight container for up to 5 days.

Tuna Salad with Capers and Olives

SERVES 4

This tuna salad is made special with a bit of Mediterranean flair. Capers and olives dress up this classic recipe to fit with your new diet.

10-12 OUNCES CANNED TUNA (1-2 CANS) IN WATER, DRAINED

¼ CUP DICED CELERY

3 TABLESPOONS FRESH LEMON JUICE

2 TABLESPOONS CHOPPED ALMONDS

2 TABLESPOONS CAPERS, RINSED AND CHOPPED

1 TABLESPOON EXTRA-VIRGIN OLIVE OIL

1 TABLESPOON CHOPPED FRESH DILL

SALT AND FRESHLY GROUND PEPPER

1. Flake the tuna with a fork into a mixing bowl.

2. Add the remaining ingredients except the salt and pepper, and stir until well combined. Season with salt and pepper.

3. Serve on toast or a bed of greens.

Three-Bean Greek Salad

SERVES 8 TO 10

Simply toss the ingredients together and you have yourself a delicious Greek salad that everyone is sure to love.

2 CUPS FROZEN GREEN BEANS, THAWED

ONE 16-OUNCE CAN KIDNEY BEANS, DRAINED AND RINSED

ONE 14.5-OUNCE CAN CUT WAX BEANS, DRAINED AND RINSED

1 CUP SLICED PITTED BLACK OLIVES

½ CUP DICED RED ONION

½ CUP DICED RED BELL PEPPER

½ CUP DICED SEEDLESS CUCUMBER

⅔ CUP STORE-BOUGHT GREEK VINAIGRETTE

1 CUP CRUMBLED FETA CHEESE

1. Combine all the ingredients except the vinaigrette and feta cheese in a mixing bowl. Toss well.

2. Drizzle the vinaigrette over the salad and toss lightly to coat. Sprinkle with feta cheese and serve.

Shaved Lamb Lettuce Wraps

SERVES 4 TO 6

A unique twist on the classic gyro, these lettuce wraps omit the cumbersome pita bread so you can better enjoy the flavor of the lamb and sauce.

2 TO 3 POUNDS ROAST LAMB, COOLED

1 HEAD BOSTON LETTUCE, RINSED WELL

½ SEEDLESS CUCUMBER, GRATED

1 CUP PLAIN NONFAT GREEK YOGURT

¼ CUP CHOPPED FRESH DILL

¼ CUP CHOPPED FRESH PARSLEY

¼ CUP CHOPPED FRESH MINT

3 TABLESPOONS FRESH LEMON JUICE

1 GARLIC CLOVE, MINCED

SALT AND FRESHLY GROUND PEPPER

2 SMALL TOMATOES, CHOPPED

½ CUP CHOPPED PEPPERONCINI

1. Remove the lamb you prepared earlier in the week from the refrigerator. Let it sit at room temperature until you are ready for it.

2. Separate the leaves from the head of lettuce and lay them flat on plates. Set aside.

3. Combine the cucumber, Greek yogurt, herbs, lemon juice, and garlic in a food processor. Blend until smooth; then season with salt and pepper.

4. Shave the lamb into thin slices using a serrated knife. Fold 1 or 2 pieces of lamb into each lettuce cup.

5. Top the lettuce with a tablespoon of sauce and serve with chopped tomatoes and pepperoncini.

Grilled Vegetable Skewers

SERVES 4 TO 6

If you are looking for something light and simple for dinner tonight, give these vegetable skewers a try.

FOR THE MARINADE:

½ CUP EXTRA-VIRGIN OLIVE OIL

½ CUP FRESH LEMON JUICE

¼ CUP WATER

3 TABLESPOONS DIJON MUSTARD

2 TABLESPOONS HONEY

1 TABLESPOON MINCED GARLIC

1 TABLESPOON CHOPPED FRESH BASIL

1 TABLESPOON CHOPPED FRESH PARSLEY

½ TEASPOON SALT

¼ TEASPOON FRESHLY GROUND PEPPER

FOR THE VEGETABLE SKEWERS:

WOODEN SKEWERS

1 RED BELL PEPPER, SEEDED AND CUT INTO 1-INCH CHUNKS

1 GREEN BELL PEPPER, SEEDED AND CUT INTO 1-INCH CHUNKS

1 RED ONION, CUT INTO 1-INCH CHUNKS

1 CUP BUTTON MUSHROOMS

1 CUP CHOPPED ZUCCHINI

1 CUP CHERRY TOMATOES

EXTRA-VIRGIN OLIVE OIL, FOR THE GRILL

To make the marinade:

Whisk all the marinade ingredients together in a small bowl. Cover and chill until ready to use.

continued ▶

To make the vegetable skewers:

1. Soak the wooden skewers in water for 30 minutes to keep them from burning on the grill.

2. Combine all the vegetables in a shallow dish. Pour the marinade over them and stir to coat.

3. Cover the vegetables and chill for 2 hours.

4. Preheat the grill to medium.

5. Brush the grates with olive oil.

6. Slide the vegetables onto the skewers and lay the skewers on the grill. Cook for 2 to 3 minutes; then turn the vegetables.

7. Baste the skewers with marinade and cook another 2 to 3 minutes before turning and basting again.

8. Cook the vegetables for a total of 10 minutes or so, turning and basting as needed, until tender. Serve hot.

Cream of Avocado Soup

SERVES 4 TO 6

Some like it hot and some like it cold. With this creamy avocado soup, you can serve it either way.

2 AVOCADOS, PEELED, PITTED, AND CHOPPED

2 TABLESPOONS FRESH LIME JUICE

2 TABLESPOONS EXTRA-VIRGIN OLIVE OIL

1 TEASPOON MINCED GARLIC

1 CUP DICED ONION

½ CUP DICED CELERY

1 SMALL JALAPEÑO, SEEDED AND MINCED

3 CUPS CHICKEN BROTH

1 CUP UNSWEETENED COCONUT MILK

SALT AND FRESHLY GROUND PEPPER

1. Toss the chopped avocados with the lime juice in a small bowl. Set aside.

2. Heat the olive oil in a stockpot over medium heat. Add the garlic and cook for 1 minute.

3. Stir in the onion, celery, and jalapeño. Cook until the onions are translucent, about 6 minutes.

4. Add 2 cups of chicken broth and bring to a boil. Reduce the heat and simmer for 10 minutes.

5. Remove the soup from heat and allow it to cool for several minutes.

6. Purée the avocado in a blender with the remaining cup of chicken broth. Add the coconut milk and blend until smooth.

7. Spoon half the mixture from the stockpot into the blender and blend smooth. Add the remaining soup and blend until well combined.

8. Season with salt and pepper. Chill if desired before serving, or serve warm.

Chopped Beet and Arugula Salad

SERVES 4

This chopped salad is unique among salads. You may not often find beets on your plate, but after trying them in this recipe, you might change your habits.

1 LARGE BEET, TRIMMED

3 TABLESPOONS ORANGE JUICE

1 TABLESPOON EXTRA-VIRGIN OLIVE OIL

1 TABLESPOON WHITE WINE VINEGAR

PINCH OF MUSTARD POWDER

SALT AND FRESHLY GROUND PEPPER

2 BUNCHES FRESH ARUGULA

2 NAVEL ORANGES, PEELED AND CHOPPED

1 CUP CRUMBLED FETA CHEESE

1. Preheat the oven to 450°F.

2. Wrap the beet in foil and place it on a baking sheet. Roast the beet for 45 to 50 minutes, or until tender.

3. Remove the beet from the oven and let cool for several minutes. Unwrap the foil and use a paper towel to rub the skin off the beet. Cut the beet into wedges and set aside.

4. For the dressing, combine the orange juice, olive oil, and white wine vinegar in a small bowl. Whisk in the mustard powder and season with salt and pepper.

5. Divide the arugula among four plates and top with the sliced beets, chopped oranges, and crumbled feta. Drizzle with the dressing to serve.

Butternut Squash Soup

SERVES 6

This squash soup is thick, creamy, and seasoned to perfection. You won't be disappointed.

4 CUPS PEELED, CHOPPED BUTTERNUT SQUASH

2 TABLESPOONS EXTRA-VIRGIN OLIVE OIL

1 TEASPOON MINCED GARLIC

½ CUP DICED CARROT

½ CUP DICED CELERY

1 MEDIUM ONION, CHOPPED

4 CUPS CHICKEN BROTH

1 TEASPOON CHOPPED FRESH THYME

SALT AND FRESHLY GROUND PEPPER

1. If you cannot find chopped butternut squash, simply purchase a large butternut squash and prepare it yourself. Cut the squash in half lengthwise and scoop out the seeds, then peel the squash and chop the flesh.

2. Heat the oil in a large stockpot over medium-high heat. Add the garlic and cook for 1 minute.

3. Stir in the carrot, celery, and onion and cook for 4 to 5 minutes, or until the onion is translucent.

4. Add the butternut squash, chicken broth, and thyme. Stir well and season with salt and pepper.

5. Bring to a boil, then reduce the heat and simmer until the squash is tender, about 30 minutes.

6. Remove the stockpot from heat and purée the soup using an immersion blender, or transfer the soup to an upright blender and purée. Serve the soup hot.

Italian-Herbed Lamb Chops

SERVES 6

Lamb chops are incredibly easy to make, and with this recipe, they have never tasted so good.

2 TABLESPOONS EXTRA-VIRGIN OLIVE OIL

1 TABLESPOON MINCED GARLIC

6 BONE-IN LAMB CHOPS, 1½ INCHES THICK

SALT AND FRESHLY GROUND PEPPER

2 TABLESPOONS WHOLE-WHEAT FLOUR

2 TABLESPOONS PLAIN BREAD CRUMBS

1 TEASPOON DRIED OREGANO

¼ TEASPOON DRIED THYME

½ TEASPOON DRIED ROSEMARY

1. Heat the olive oil and garlic in a heavy skillet over medium-low heat.

2. Season the lamb chops with salt and pepper.

3. Combine the flour, bread crumbs, and herbs in a shallow dish and dredge the lamb chops to coat.

4. Arrange the chops in the skillet and cook for 5 to 7 minutes on each side, or until lightly browned, flipping every 3 minutes.

5. Let the chops rest in the skillet for 3 to 4 minutes before serving.

Mediterranean Chicken Stew

SERVES 4

This chicken stew combines some of the best Mediterranean flavors. Not only do you get a hint of olive oil and garlic, but you also get to enjoy whole tomatoes and escarole.

1½ TABLESPOONS EXTRA-VIRGIN OLIVE OIL
1½ POUNDS BONELESS SKINLESS CHICKEN, CHOPPED
SALT AND FRESHLY GROUND PEPPER
1 TABLESPOON MINCED GARLIC
1 MEDIUM ONION, SLICED THIN
½ TEASPOON DRIED OREGANO
ONE 28-OUNCE CAN WHOLE PEELED TOMATOES
2 MEDIUM HEADS ESCAROLE, TRIMMED AND CHOPPED
2 CUPS WHOLE-WHEAT COUSCOUS, COOKED

1. Heat the oil in a heavy stockpot over medium-high heat.

2. Season the chicken with salt and pepper; then add it to the stockpot. Cook the chicken for 5 minutes, stirring often, until it's lightly browned.

3. Transfer the chicken to a plate; then add the garlic and onion to the stockpot. Stir in the oregano and season with salt and pepper. Cook for 3 to 4 minutes, or until the onion begins to brown.

4. Stir in the tomatoes and cook for 10 minutes, breaking the tomatoes up with a wooden spoon as you stir.

5. Add the chicken back to the pot and bring it to a simmer. Cover and cook the stew for 2 to 4 minutes, or until the chicken is cooked through.

6. Stir in the escarole and cook, stirring, until tender, 2 to 4 minutes.

7. Serve the stew hot over cooked couscous.

Goat Cheese–Stuffed Tomatoes

SERVES 6

These stuffed tomatoes are perfect for a light meal or they can double as appetizers for your next dinner party.

6 MEDIUM TOMATOES

2 CUPS COOKED QUINOA

3 OUNCES GOAT CHEESE CRUMBLES

2 TABLESPOONS CHOPPED FRESH BASIL

2 TABLESPOONS CHOPPED FRESH PARSLEY

SALT AND FRESHLY GROUND PEPPER

2 TABLESPOONS GRATED PARMESAN CHEESE

1. Preheat the oven to 350°F.

2. Lightly grease a glass baking dish.

3. Using a sharp knife, slice the tops off the tomatoes and scoop out the pulp. Discard the pulp and set the tomatoes upside down on paper towels to drain.

4. Meanwhile, combine the quinoa, goat cheese, and herbs in a mixing bowl. Season with salt and pepper.

5. Spoon the quinoa mixture into the tomatoes and arrange them in the baking dish. Sprinkle the quinoa mixture with the Parmesan cheese.

6. Bake the tomatoes for 15 to 20 minutes, or until tender. Serve hot.

Maple Lime Salmon

SERVES 4

If you are a fan of salmon but don't like it breaded or fried, this recipe is perfect for you. A hint of maple and lime serve to enhance the salmon without covering up its delicious flavor.

ONE 1½-POUND SALMON FILLET, 1-INCH THICK
SALT
1 TABLESPOON MAPLE SYRUP
2 LIMES

1. Preheat the oven to 450°F.

2. Remove any visible bones from the fillet.

3. Sprinkle a baking sheet with salt and place the fillet on the baking sheet, skin-side down.

4. Drizzle the maple syrup over the salmon and sprinkle with salt.

5. Zest the limes and sprinkle the zest over the salmon fillet.

6. Bake the salmon fillet for 10 to 15 minutes, or until the salmon flakes easily with a fork.

7. Squeeze the lime juice over the fillet to serve.

Broiled Turkey Burgers with Arugula

SERVES 4

These broiled turkey burgers couldn't be easier. Simply combine the ingredients, shape them into patties, and throw them in the oven.

1 POUND LEAN GROUND TURKEY

1 CUP CRUMBLED FETA CHEESE

¼ CUP DICED RED ONION

1 TABLESPOON CHOPPED FRESH DILL

1 GARLIC CLOVE, MINCED

1 TABLESPOON DIJON MUSTARD

1 TEASPOON WHITE WINE VINEGAR

½ TEASPOON BALSAMIC VINEGAR

PINCH OF SALT

PINCH OF FRESHLY GROUND PEPPER

4 WHOLE-GRAIN SANDWICH BUNS

2 CUPS FRESH ARUGULA

1. Preheat the broiler to high heat.

2. Combine the turkey, feta, onion, dill, and garlic in a mixing bowl. Mix it well by hand; then shape the turkey mixture into 4 matching patties.

3. Place the patties on a broiler pan and slide it under the broiler. Broil for 4 to 5 minutes on each side, or until cooked through.

4. Whisk together the mustard, vinegars, salt, and pepper in a small bowl.

5. Toast the sandwich buns, if desired.

6. Spread a thin layer of the mustard mixture on the top half of each bun.

7. Place a cooked turkey burger on the bottom half of each bun and top with about ½ cup of fresh arugula. Top with the other half of the bun to serve.

Winter Vegetable Ragout

SERVES 4

If you don't have much time to prepare dinner in the evening, give this vegetable ragout a try. Simply combine the ingredients in the morning and come home to a fully cooked meal.

2 TABLESPOONS EXTRA-VIRGIN OLIVE OIL

1 TABLESPOON MINCED GARLIC

1 POUND SMALL RED POTATOES, CHOPPED

1 CUP BABY CARROTS

4 MEDIUM SHALLOTS, PEELED AND HALVED

2 SMALL TURNIPS, PEELED AND CHOPPED

1½ CUPS VEGETABLE BROTH

¼ CUP DRY WHITE WINE

1 TABLESPOON CHOPPED FRESH SAGE

½ TEASPOON DRIED THYME

SALT AND FRESHLY GROUND PEPPER

1. Combine the oil and garlic in the bottom of a slow cooker. Add the vegetables and toss to coat.

2. Stir in the vegetable broth, wine, sage, and thyme. Season with salt and pepper.

3. Cover the slow cooker and cook on low heat for 6 to 8 hours, or until the vegetables are tender. Serve hot.

Lemon-Basil Shrimp and Linguine

SERVES 4

This shrimp with linguine is so simple, you may not believe it. Just because it is easy to prepare, however, doesn't mean it doesn't pack a punch with delicious flavor.

FOR THE SHRIMP:
JUICE FROM 1 LEMON
½ CUP CHOPPED FRESH BASIL
SALT AND FRESHLY GROUND PEPPER
1 POUND RAW SHRIMP, PEELED AND DEVEINED

FOR THE LINGUINE:
SALT
12 OUNCES WHOLE-WHEAT LINGUINE
1 TABLESPOON EXTRA-VIRGIN OLIVE OIL
1 TABLESPOON MINCED GARLIC
1 MEDIUM TOMATO, CHOPPED

To make the shrimp:

1. Whisk together the lemon juice and basil in a small bowl and season with salt and pepper.

2. Arrange the shrimp in a shallow dish and pour the marinade over them. Toss well to coat the shrimp and chill them for 20 minutes.

To make the linguine:

1. Bring a large pot of salted water to a rolling boil. Add the linguine and cook al dente according to the package directions. Drain the linguine and set aside.

2. Heat the olive oil in a large skillet over medium heat. Add the garlic and cook for 1 minute.

3. Stir in the tomato and cook for 2 to 3 minutes longer.

4. Add the marinated shrimp and stir well. Cover the skillet and cook for 2 to 3 minutes, or until the shrimp are pink.

5. Stir in the cooked linguine and cook until just heated through. Serve hot.

Dessert Recipes

Simple Lemon Sorbet

SERVES 6 TO 8

If you are looking for a simple yet refreshing dessert, try out this lemon sorbet.

1 CUP WATER
¾ CUP SUGAR
¾ CUP FRESH LEMON JUICE

1. Whisk together the water and sugar in a saucepan over medium heat. Stir until the sugar dissolves. Remove the sugar water from the heat and set aside.

2. Whisk in the lemon juice, then cover the mixture and chill it until cold.

3. Pour the mixture into a shallow pan and freeze it for 1 hour. Stir the mixture, then refreeze it until it is solid.

4. Just before serving, break the sorbet into pieces and blend it smooth in a food processor.

Chocolate-Covered Figs

MAKES 24 FIGS

Chocolate-covered figs have just the right amount of sweet and chocolate flavor, plus a little almond crunch.

½ CUP CHOPPED ALMONDS
1¼ CUPS SEMISWEET CHOCOLATE CHIPS
24 DRIED FIGS

1. Line a baking sheet with parchment paper and set aside.

2. Place the almonds in a shallow dish and set aside.

3. Melt the chocolate chips in a double boiler over medium-low heat, stirring until the chocolate is smooth and melted.

4. Hold the figs by the stem and dip them, one at a time, into the melted chocolate.

5. Let the excess chocolate drip off; then dip the figs in the chopped almonds and set them on the parchment-lined baking sheet.

6. Set aside to cool for 2 hours, or until the chocolate hardens. Store in an airtight container in the refrigerator for up to 3 days.

Spiced Rice Pudding

SERVES 4

Rice pudding is a unique dessert that you may not have tried before. It is worth making at least once, however, because that is all it will take to make you fall in love with it.

2½ CUPS SKIM MILK

⅓ CUP UNCOOKED WHITE RICE

PINCH OF SALT

1 EGG

¼ CUP PACKED BROWN SUGAR

1 TEASPOON VANILLA EXTRACT

⅓ CUP RAISINS

⅛ TEASPOON GROUND CINNAMON

⅛ TEASPOON GROUND NUTMEG

1. Bring the milk, rice, and salt to boil in a medium saucepan over high heat.

2. Reduce the heat to low and simmer for 20 to 25 minutes, or until the rice is tender, stirring frequently.

3. Beat together the egg and brown sugar in a mixing bowl. Stir in ½ cup of hot rice, 1 tablespoon at a time, and stir well.

4. Pour the egg mixture into the saucepan and stir over low heat for about 8 minutes, until thickened. Do not boil.

5. Remove the mixture from the heat, then stir in the raisins, vanilla extract, cinnamon, and nutmeg to serve.

Peanut Butter Oatmeal Balls

These treats don't require any baking. In fact, they take hardly any preparation at all.

1 CUP OLD-FASHIONED OATS

½ CUP GROUND FLAXSEED

¼ CUP SMOOTH PEANUT BUTTER

¼ CUP SMOOTH ALMOND BUTTER

3 TABLESPOONS HONEY

1 TABLESPOON CHIA SEEDS

½ TEASPOON GROUND CINNAMON

PINCH OF SALT

1. Combine all the ingredients in a bowl. Stir until well combined.

2. Roll the dough into 1-inch balls by hand and arrange them on a plate. Refrigerate until firm, about 1 hour.

Strawberry Almond Smoothie

SERVES 2

This smoothie is the ultimate in simple desserts. Simply throw the ingredients together in a blender to make this quick treat.

2 CUPS FROZEN STRAWBERRIES
1 CUP UNSWEETENED ALMOND MILK
½ CUP ICE CUBES
2 TABLESPOONS ALMOND BUTTER

1. Combine all the ingredients in a blender and blend on high speed until smooth and combined.

2. Pour the smoothie into two glasses and serve immediately.

Honey-Glazed Almonds

MAKES 2 CUPS

These glazed almonds are sure to satisfy your sweet tooth. Sweet and crunchy, they may become a new favorite.

2 CUPS WHOLE ALMONDS
2 TABLESPOONS HONEY
2 TABLESPOONS WATER
2 TABLESPOONS CANOLA OIL
PINCH OF SALT

1. Preheat the oven to 350°F.

2. Spread the almonds in a rimmed baking sheet and bake for 10 minutes, or until they are lightly toasted.

3. Combine the honey, water, and canola oil in a heavy skillet over medium heat. Bring the mixture to a boil, then stir in the almonds.

4. Cook the almonds for 3 minutes, or until the liquid evaporates.

5. Stir in the salt and cook until the almonds are reddish brown. Remove the almonds from the heat.

6. Spread the almonds on parchment paper to cool before serving.

Cinnamon-Walnut Biscotti

SERVES 12

These biscotti have just the right amount of crunch, not to mention a great deal of flavor.

1¼ CUPS WHOLE-WHEAT FLOUR

⅓ CUP SUGAR

1 TEASPOON BAKING POWDER

PINCH OF SALT

½ CUP CHOPPED WALNUTS

¼ CUP RAISINS

2 EGGS

1 TEASPOON VANILLA EXTRACT

1 TEASPOON SKIM MILK

1. Preheat the oven to 350°F.

2. Line a rimmed baking sheet with parchment paper.

3. Whisk together the flour, sugar, baking powder, and salt in a mixing bowl. Fold in the walnuts and raisins.

4. In another bowl, beat together the eggs, vanilla extract, and skim milk.

5. Add the wet ingredients to the dry, stirring until just combined.

6. Turn the dough onto a floured surface and roll it into a rectangular loaf.

7. Place the loaf on the baking sheet and bake for 25 minutes, or until it rises. Cool the loaf on a wire rack for 1 hour.

8. Reheat the oven to 300°F.

9. Move the loaf to a cutting board and slice it into ¼-inch-thick slices. Arrange the slices on the baking sheet.

10. Bake the slices for 15 minutes, then flip them and bake for another 10 to 15 minutes, or until they are crisp and lightly browned. Cool the biscotti completely before serving.

CHAPTER FOUR

Week Two

The Mediterranean diet has been under research for over 50 years, and its benefits continue to become apparent . . . The good news is that you do not need to live in this geographic area to get these benefits. All that you need to do is understand where they come from and what changes you can make to your diet to get them.

—Betty Kovacs, MedicineNet.com

WEEK TWO MEAL PLAN

Day One

Breakfast: Cranberry Almond Oatmeal
Lunch: Simple Mediterranean Salad
Dinner: Steamed Mussels in Garlic Wine Broth
Snacks: 1 cup chopped watermelon; ⅛ ounce sliced avocado
Dessert: Strawberry Banana Tart

> **Daily Tip:** Try using lavender oil to ease stress and relax. Place a few drops in a hot bath and soak for a while before bed.

Day Two

Breakfast: Mushroom and Red Onion Omelet
Lunch: Roasted Vegetable Panini
Dinner: Stuffed Bell Peppers
Snacks: 30 shelled pistachios; 1 small apple
Dessert: Spiced Pecans

> **Daily Tip:** Don't be ashamed to get a monthly massage. Deep tissue massages can help with issues like back pain and more.

Day Three

Breakfast: Chocolate Zucchini Muffins
Lunch: Artichoke and Feta Couscous
Dinner: Hearty Beef and Sweet Potato Stew
Snacks: 1 scoop nonfat frozen yogurt; 1 small orange
Dessert: Maple Grilled Peaches

> Garlic is known for its antiviral and antibacterial properties, but recent studies suggest that it may also help ward off cancer.

Day Four

Breakfast: Orange-Hempseed Smoothie
Lunch: Curried Acorn Squash Soup
Dinner: Pan-Seared Scallops with Steamed Vegetables
Snacks: 3 dark chocolate squares; 3 tablespoons dried fruit
Dessert: Blueberry Lime Sorbet

> **Daily Tip:** Try to shake up your exercise routine a little bit. Do something new once or twice a week to keep from getting bored.

Day Five

Breakfast: Spiced Pumpkin Bread
Lunch: Lemon Orzo Tuna Salad
Dinner: Lemon Caper Chicken
Snacks: 2 tablespoons hummus with 8 baby carrots; ½ small banana
Dessert: Cranberry Almond Biscotti

Daily Tip: Avocados are rich in monounsaturated fats and vitamin E. Enjoy a slice for a snack or use it as a salad topper.

Day Six

Breakfast: Scallion Scrambled Eggs
Lunch: Whole-Grain Mediterranean Pizza
Dinner: Stuffed Portobello Mushroom Caps
Snacks: 1 cup fresh blueberries; ½ ounce turkey jerky
Dessert: Apple Cinnamon Scones

Daily Tip: If you want to build muscle, lift heavier weights for fewer repetitions.

Day Seven

Breakfast: Cranberry Walnut Granola
Lunch: Arugula Cucumber Mint Salad
Dinner: Baked Halibut with Mango Salsa
Snacks: ½ cup fruit salad; 3 cups air-popped popcorn
Dessert: Chocolate Bread Pudding

Daily Tip: Keep your mind sharp by engaging in conversation daily with coworkers and family. You might also try doing a crossword puzzle to get your brain going.

Note: The snacks included in this meal plan are simple snacks you can purchase from the grocery store that need little to no preparation. For more information regarding the nutritional content of these snacks, refer to Appendix A.

ADDITIONAL TIPS FOR WEEK TWO:

- Dehydration is a common trigger of headaches, and it can also contribute to migraines. To protect yourself, drink plenty of water each day. You may even want to start carrying a bottle of water with you.
- If you are trying to reduce belly fat, keep an eye on your carbohydrate intake. You don't need to skimp, but be sure you are getting enough protein in your diet to balance the carbs.
- Cayenne pepper has been shown to increase blood flow and circulation. Sprinkle a little on your meal to enjoy the flavor and benefits.

WEEK TWO SHOPPING LIST

To prepare your meals for this week, purchase the following items in the quantities indicated:

Pantry Items

- Cayenne pepper
- Cinnamon, ground
- Cloves, ground
- Cumin, ground
- Curry powder
- Nutmeg, ground
- Oregano, dried
- Pepper
- Pumpkin pie spice
- Salt
- Canola oil
- Coconut oil
- Cooking spray
- Olive oil, extra-virgin
- Almond extract
- Vanilla extract
- Baking powder
- Baking soda
- Cocoa powder, unsweetened
- Vinegar, balsamic
- Vinegar, red wine
- Soy sauce
- Honey
- Maple syrup
- Garlic

Produce

- Basil (1 bunch)
- Chives (1 bunch)
- Cilantro (1 bunch)
- Mint (1 bunch)
- Parsley (1 bunch)
- Thyme (1 bunch)
- Apple (1 medium)
- Bananas (2)
- Cherries, pitted (2 cups)
- Lemons (3)
- Limes (1)
- Mango (1)
- Oranges, navel (3)
- Peaches (4)
- Strawberries (2 cups)
- Arugula (4 cups)
- Bell peppers, red (5)
- Broccoli (1 bunch)
- Carrots, baby (1 cup)
- Cauliflower florets (2 cups)
- Cucumbers, seedless (2 small)
- Eggplant (1 medium)
- Lettuce, romaine (1 head)
- Onion, red (1 small)
- Onions (2 medium)
- Potatoes, sweet (3 medium)
- Radishes (4 small)
- Scallions (2 bunches)

- Shallots (2 medium)
- Tomatoes (5)
- Squash, acorn (3 medium)
- Zucchini (2 medium)
- Mushrooms, button (4 cups)
- Mushrooms, portobello (6 large)

Protein

- Beef chuck roast (1¼ pounds)
- Chicken breast halves, skinless (four, 4 ounces)
- Halibut fillets (four, 4 to 6 ounces)
- Mussels, live (4 pounds)
- Scallops, large (1½ pounds)
- Tuna, canned in water (two 12-ounce cans)

Dairy

- Butter (6 tablespoons)
- Coconut milk, unsweetened (1 cup)
- Milk, skim (1½ cups)
- Feta cheese, crumbled (4¾ cups)
- Mozzarella cheese, shredded (1 cup)
- Parmesan cheese, grated (¾ cup)
- Provolone cheese (4 slices)
- Yogurt, plain nonfat Greek (1¾ cups)

Dry Foods

- Flour, unbleached (3 cups)
- Flour, whole-wheat (7 cups)
- Yeast, instant (2 teaspoons)
- Sugar (3 cups)
- Sugar, brown (½ cup)
- Bread crumbs, plain (¼ cup)
- Couscous, whole-wheat (2¼ cups)
- Hempseed (1 tablespoon)
- Oats, old-fashioned (2 cups)
- Oats, rolled (1 cup)
- Oats, steel-cut (1 cup)
- Pasta, orzo (12 ounces)
- Beans, white cannellini (one 15-ounce can)
- Apricots, dried (½ cup)
- Cranberries, dried (1¼ cups)
- Raisins, golden (½ cup)
- Almonds, chopped (½ cups)
- Almonds, slivered (1¼ cups)
- Almonds, toasted and chopped (¼ cup)
- Pecans, whole (4 cups)
- Walnuts, chopped (¼ cup)

Refrigerated and Frozen Foods

- Eggs (23)
- Orange juice (1¼ cups)

- Blueberries, frozen (4 cups)
- Spinach, frozen (10 ounces)

Other

- Bread, ciabatta (1 loaf)
- Bread, whole-grain (1 loaf)
- Artichoke hearts, marinated (three 6-ounce jars)
- Black olives, pitted (1¾ cups)
- Capers (2 tablespoons)
- Chocolate chips, mini (½ cup)
- Pizza sauce (¼ cup)
- Pumpkin purée (2 cups)

- Sun-dried tomatoes in oil (½ cup)
- Sherry, dry (⅓ cup)
- Tomatoes, diced (one 14.5-ounce can)
- White wine, dry (2 cups)
- Broth, beef (1½ cups)
- Broth, chicken (3 cups)
- Broth, vegetable (1½ cups)

PLAN-AHEAD PREPARATIONS

This week there are several things you can prepare ahead of time and use throughout the week to make your life easier.

1. **Sliced black olives:** You will use these in several recipes. If you prefer not to buy pre-sliced olives, purchase them whole and slice them yourself using a small, sharp knife.
2. **Fresh lemon juice:** Lemon juice will be used in several recipes this week. Juice several lemons at a time and store the juice in an airtight container in the fridge.
3. **Beef stew meat:** To cut your own beef stew meat for your Hearty Beef and Sweet Potato Stew, start with a 1¾-pound boneless beef chuck roast. Trim the fat from the roast and cut the meat into 1-inch chunks.
4. **Whole-grain pizza crust:** Because the pizza crust in the Whole-Grain Mediterranean Pizza recipe takes several hours to set and rise, you may need to prepare it the day before so you can just top the pizza and cook it when you are ready to eat.

WEEK TWO RECIPES

Breakfast Recipes

CRANBERRY ALMOND OATMEAL

MUSHROOM AND RED ONION OMELET

CHOCOLATE ZUCCHINI MUFFINS

ORANGE-HEMPSEED SMOOTHIE

SPICED PUMPKIN BREAD

SCALLION SCRAMBLED EGGS

CRANBERRY WALNUT GRANOLA

Lunch Recipes

SIMPLE MEDITERRANEAN SALAD

ROASTED VEGETABLE PANINI

ARTICHOKE AND FETA COUSCOUS

CURRIED ACORN SQUASH SOUP

LEMON ORZO TUNA SALAD

WHOLE-GRAIN MEDITERRANEAN PIZZA

ARUGULA CUCUMBER MINT SALAD

Dinner Recipes

STEAMED MUSSELS IN GARLIC WINE BROTH

STUFFED BELL PEPPERS

HEARTY BEEF AND SWEET POTATO STEW

PAN-SEARED SCALLOPS WITH STEAMED VEGGIES

LEMON CAPER CHICKEN

STUFFED PORTOBELLO MUSHROOM CAPS

BAKED HALIBUT WITH MANGO SALSA

Dessert Recipes

STRAWBERRY BANANA TART

SPICED PECANS

MAPLE GRILLED PEACHES

BLUEBERRY LIME SORBET

CRANBERRY ALMOND BISCOTTI

APPLE CINNAMON SCONES

CHOCOLATE BREAD PUDDING

Cranberry Almond Oatmeal

SERVES 4

Oatmeal is a morning staple in many families, but it can get boring after a while. Shake things up with this cranberry and almond version.

2 CUPS WATER

1 CUP STEEL-CUT OATS

⅓ CUP DRIED CRANBERRIES

¼ TEASPOON GROUND CINNAMON

PINCH OF SALT

¼ CUP SLIVERED ALMONDS

1 TABLESPOON MAPLE SYRUP

1. Whisk together the water and steel-cut oats in a small saucepan over medium-heat.

2. Add the cranberries, cinnamon, and salt.

3. Bring to a boil, then reduce the heat and simmer on low, uncovered, for about 20 minutes.

4. Spoon the oatmeal into bowls and top with slivered almonds and a drizzle of maple syrup to serve.

Mushroom and Red Onion Omelet

SERVES 2

This filling omelet is the perfect way to start your day. Full of the flavors of tender mushrooms and fresh red onions, this omelet will keep you satisfied all morning long.

2 EGGS

1 TABLESPOON SKIM MILK

½ TEASPOON SALT

¼ TEASPOON FRESHLY GROUND PEPPER

2 TEASPOONS EXTRA-VIRGIN OLIVE OIL

1 CUP CHOPPED BUTTON MUSHROOMS

3 TABLESPOONS DICED RED ONION

1. Crack the eggs into a small bowl and whisk in the skim milk, salt, and pepper until well combined. Set the bowl aside.

2. Heat 1 teaspoon of olive oil in a small skillet over medium heat.

3. Add the mushrooms and red onion to the skillet and cook for 2 to 3 minutes, or until hot.

4. Spoon the mushroom mixture into a bowl and set aside.

5. Heat the remaining teaspoon of olive oil in the same skillet and pour in the egg mixture. Rotate the pan to coat the sides with egg.

6. Let the eggs cook for 1 minute; then scrape down the sides of the pan using a spatula, letting the uncooked eggs spread.

7. Allow the eggs to cook for 1 to 2 minutes longer, or until almost set. Spoon the mushroom mixture over half of the omelet.

8. Fold the empty half of the omelet over the mushroom filling and allow the eggs to cook for 1 more minute, or until the eggs are cooked through. Serve hot.

Chocolate Zucchini Muffins

MAKES 12 MUFFINS

These muffins walk the fine line between breakfast pastry and dessert. You won't be thinking about that, however, when you are digging in.

1 CUP GRATED ZUCCHINI

1 CUP ROLLED OATS

1 CUP WHOLE-WHEAT FLOUR

2 TABLESPOONS UNSWEETENED COCOA POWDER

1 TEASPOON GROUND CINNAMON

1 TEASPOON BAKING SODA

½ TEASPOON SALT

½ CUP HONEY

2 EGGS

1 TEASPOON VANILLA EXTRACT

1. Preheat the oven to 325°F.

2. Place the grated zucchini in a clean dish towel and wring as much moisture from it as possible.

3. Combine the oats, flour, cocoa powder, cinnamon, baking soda, and salt in a medium mixing bowl and stir well.

4. In a separate mixing bowl, beat the honey, eggs, and vanilla extract until smooth.

5. Add the dry ingredients to the wet ingredients in small batches, stirring until smooth after each addition.

6. Fold in the grated zucchini until just combined.

7. Line a muffin tin with paper liners and fill each cup about two-thirds full with batter.

8. Bake the muffins for 20 to 25 minutes, or until a knife inserted in the center comes out clean.

9. Cool the muffins in the pan for 5 minutes; then turn the muffins out onto a wire cooling rack to cool completely before serving.

Orange-Hempseed Smoothie

SERVES 2

Hempseed is a good source of vegetarian protein, which is just what this smoothie needs.

2 NAVEL ORANGES, PEELED AND CHOPPED

1 CUP ORANGE JUICE

1 CUP PLAIN NONFAT GREEK YOGURT

½ CUP ICE CUBES

1 TABLESPOON HEMPSEED

1. Combine the chopped oranges and orange juice in a blender. Blend until smooth.

2. Add the remaining ingredients and blend on high speed for 1 minute. Pour the smoothie into two glasses and serve immediately.

Spiced Pumpkin Bread

MAKES 1 LOAF

Though it is listed as a breakfast recipe here, you may enjoy this pumpkin bread all day long. Try it out for a snack or even dessert.

COOKING SPRAY
2 CUPS PUMPKIN PURÉE
½ CUP CANOLA OIL
2 EGGS
1 CUP SUGAR
¼ CUP SKIM MILK
¾ TEASPOON VANILLA EXTRACT
1 CUP WHOLE-WHEAT FLOUR
1 CUP UNBLEACHED FLOUR
1 TEASPOON BAKING SODA
½ TEASPOON BAKING POWDER
½ TEASPOON SALT
1½ TEASPOONS PUMPKIN PIE SPICE

1. Preheat the oven to 350°F.

2. Lightly grease a standard loaf pan with cooking spray.

3. Whisk together the pumpkin purée, canola oil, eggs, sugar, milk, and vanilla extract in a large mixing bowl.

4. In a separate bowl, stir together the flours, baking soda, baking powder, salt, and pumpkin pie spice.

5. Stir the dry ingredients into the wet ingredients until the mixture is well combined.

6. Spoon the batter into the prepared pan and bake for 60 to 75 minutes, or until a knife inserted in the center of the loaf comes out clean.

7. Remove the loaf from the oven and let it stand for 10 minutes. Turn the loaf out onto a wire rack to cool completely before cutting.

Scallion Scrambled Eggs

SERVES 2

These scrambled eggs are a great option if you are in need of a quick and simple morning meal.

4 EGGS

1 TABLESPOON SKIM MILK

1 TEASPOON EXTRA-VIRGIN OLIVE OIL

1 TEASPOON MINCED GARLIC

¼ CUP SLICED SCALLIONS

SALT AND FRESHLY GROUND PEPPER

1. Whisk together the eggs and skim milk in a small bowl and set aside.

2. Heat the olive oil in a small skillet over medium-high heat. Add the garlic and cook for 1 minute.

3. Stir in the egg mixture and tilt the pan to coat it evenly. Cook for 30 seconds without stirring.

4. Stirring slowly to scramble the eggs into chunks, let the egg cook for 2 to 3 minutes, or until set.

5. Stir in the scallions, season with salt and pepper, and serve.

Cranberry Walnut Granola

SERVES 6

This nutty granola is sure to give your mornings a crunch.

2 CUPS OLD-FASHIONED OATS
⅓ CUP SLIVERED ALMONDS
¼ CUP CHOPPED WALNUTS
1 TEASPOON GROUND CINNAMON
PINCH OF SALT
3 TABLESPOONS CANOLA OIL
¼ CUP HONEY
¼ CUP PACKED BROWN SUGAR
1 TEASPOON VANILLA EXTRACT
½ CUP DRIED CRANBERRIES

1. Preheat the oven to 375°F.

2. Line a rimmed baking sheet with parchment paper.

3. Combine the old-fashioned oats, almonds, and walnuts in a large mixing bowl with the cinnamon and salt. Toss well.

4. In a small bowl, whisk together the canola oil, honey, brown sugar, and vanilla extract.

5. Pour the canola oil mixture over the oat mixture and mix well by hand until the oats are coated. Spread the oat mixture out on the prepared baking sheet.

6. Bake for 10 minutes; then turn the granola with a spatula and bake 5 to 10 minutes more, or until just browned.

7. Transfer the mixture to a large bowl to cool and toss with the dried cranberries. Store in an airtight container for up to 5 days.

Simple Mediterranean Salad

SERVES 8

This simple salad combines classic Greek flavors like olives, tomato, feta, and red wine vinegar. Try it once and you're sure to try it again.

1 HEAD ROMAINE LETTUCE, CHOPPED

4 TOMATOES, CUT INTO WEDGES

1 SEEDLESS CUCUMBER, DICED

½ RED ONION, SLICED THIN

1 CUP PITTED BLACK OLIVES, PLUS 2 TABLESPOONS MINCED

1 CUP CRUMBLED FETA CHEESE

¼ CUP EXTRA-VIRGIN OLIVE OIL

2 TABLESPOONS RED WINE VINEGAR

1 TEASPOON HONEY

1 TEASPOON MINCED GARLIC

SALT AND FRESHLY GROUND PEPPER

1. Combine the lettuce, tomatoes, cucumber, onions, and 1 cup of olives in a bowl. Stir to combine. Toss with ½ cup of feta cheese.

2. Whisk together the olive oil, red wine vinegar, honey, garlic, and 2 tablespoons of minced black olives in a small bowl. Season with salt and pepper.

3. Pour the olive oil mixture over the salad and toss to coat.

4. Toss the salad with the remaining ½ cup of feta cheese to serve.

Roasted Vegetable Panini

SERVES 4

This vegetarian panini gives you the satisfaction of enjoying a hearty lunch without the extra calories or saturated fat of lunch meat.

1 TABLESPOON EXTRA-VIRGIN OLIVE OIL

2 TABLESPOONS BALSAMIC VINEGAR

SALT AND FRESHLY GROUND PEPPER

COOKING SPRAY

1 MEDIUM EGGPLANT, CUT INTO ¼-INCH SLICES

1 MEDIUM ZUCCHINI, CUT INTO ¼-INCH SLICES

1 RED BELL PEPPER, SEEDED AND SLICED

8 SLICES CIABATTA BREAD

4 SLICES PROVOLONE CHEESE

8 FRESH BASIL LEAVES

1. Preheat the broiler.

2. Whisk together the olive oil and vinegar in a small bowl. Season the mixture with salt and pepper.

3. Grease a baking sheet with cooking spray and spread the vegetables on it. Brush the vegetables with the half of the olive oil mixture.

4. Broil the vegetables for 7 to 8 minutes, turning once.

5. Brush the slices of ciabatta bread with the remaining olive oil mixture. Top half the slices with roasted veggies.

6. Divide the cheese and basil leaves among the sandwiches and top each with another slice of bread.

7. Heat a nonstick skillet over medium-high heat and grease it lightly with cooking spray. Add the sandwiches and cook for 2 to 3 minutes on each side, pressing flat with a spatula. Serve immediately.

Artichoke and Feta Couscous

SERVES 4 TO 6

This simple dish is a combination of heart-healthy ingredients, including arti-choke hearts and olive oil.

2 CUPS WATER

½ CUP SUN-DRIED TOMATOES IN OIL, DRAINED

1½ CUPS VEGETABLE BROTH

1¾ CUPS UNCOOKED WHOLE-WHEAT COUSCOUS

½ CUP CRUMBLED FETA CHEESE

1 CUP CHOPPED FRESH PARSLEY

TWO 6-OUNCE JARS MARINATED ARTICHOKE HEARTS, DRAINED, RINSED
    AND QUARTERED

SALT AND FRESHLY GROUND PEPPER

1. Combine the water and sun-dried tomatoes in a small saucepan and bring to a boil. Turn off the heat and let stand until the tomatoes are soft; then drain and chop the tomatoes.

2. In a large saucepan, bring the vegetable broth to boil. Stir in the couscous, cover, and reduce the heat to low. Simmer for 8 minutes, or until the couscous is tender.

3. Remove the couscous from the heat and stir in the tomatoes and the remaining ingredients to serve.

Curried Acorn Squash Soup

SERVES 4 TO 6

This soup is a recipe you will be glad to have when it gets cold. Don't be afraid to enjoy it during other seasons, too.

3 MEDIUM ACORN SQUASH

2 TABLESPOONS EXTRA-VIRGIN OLIVE OIL

½ CUP CHOPPED ONION

1 TABLESPOON CURRY POWDER

3 CUPS CHICKEN BROTH

1 CUP UNSWEETENED COCONUT MILK

½ TEASPOON GROUND NUTMEG

SALT AND FRESHLY GROUND PEPPER

1. Preheat the oven to 350°F.

2. Cut the acorn squash in half and scoop out the seeds. Place the squash cut-side down on a baking sheet.

3. Bake the squash for 35 to 40 minutes, or until just tender.

4. Heat the oil in a saucepan over medium heat. Add the onion and curry powder and cook for 4 to 6 minutes, or until the onions are tender. Remove the onion from heat and set aside.

5. Scoop the squash out of the skins and into the saucepan. Stir in the broth in small amounts until smooth.

6. Return the saucepan to medium heat and simmer for 15 to 20 minutes.

7. Allow the soup to cool slightly; then blend the soup in a food processor until smooth and return it to the pan.

8. Whisk in the coconut milk and nutmeg, season with salt and pepper, and cook until heated through.

Lemon Orzo Tuna Salad

SERVES 4

If you are looking for a recipe that is light and fresh, this tuna salad is certainly one to try.

12 OUNCES UNCOOKED ORZO PASTA

1 CUP SLICED SCALLIONS

½ CUP GOLDEN RAISINS

⅓ CUP EXTRA-VIRGIN OLIVE OIL

¼ CUP FRESH LEMON JUICE

1 TABLESPOON LEMON ZEST

SALT AND FRESHLY GROUND PEPPER

TWO 12-OUNCE CANS TUNA IN WATER, DRAINED

1. Cook the orzo according to the package directions, and drain.

2. Place the orzo in a bowl and toss with the remaining ingredients. Season with salt and pepper, and serve.

Whole-Grain Mediterranean Pizza

MAKES 12 TO 16 SLICES

This whole-grain pizza is fairly easy to put together, though it does take some time. You will need to prepare the crust a day ahead so you can cook it when you are ready to eat.

FOR THE CRUST:

3 CUPS WHOLE-WHEAT FLOUR

2 TEASPOONS INSTANT YEAST

2 TABLESPOONS HONEY

2 TABLESPOONS ORANGE JUICE

2 TABLESPOONS EXTRA-VIRGIN OLIVE OIL

¾ CUP WARM WATER

1 TEASPOON SALT

FOR THE TOPPING:

2 TABLESPOONS EXTRA-VIRGIN OLIVE OIL

¼ CUP PIZZA SAUCE

1 TOMATO, SLICED THIN

1 CUP CHOPPED MARINATED ARTICHOKE HEARTS,
    DRAINED AND RINSED

½ CUP SLICED BLACK OLIVES

1 CUP SHREDDED MOZZARELLA

1 CUP CRUMBLED FETA CHEESE

2 TABLESPOONS GRATED PARMESAN CHEESE

To make the crust:

1. Combine all the crust ingredients in a bowl and stir well. Let the mixture rest for 30 minutes.

2. Knead the mixture by hand into a soft dough, then transfer the dough to a bowl and cover. Let the dough sit for 30 minutes at room temperature.

3. Chill the dough for 18 hours or overnight.

4. Pat the dough into a lightly greased half-sheet pan.

To make the topping:

1. To prepare the pizza, brush the crust with olive oil and cover it with the pizza sauce.

2. Top the sauce with the vegetables, then cover and let the dough rise for 2 hours, or until the dough is puffy.

3. Combine the cheeses in a bowl and set aside.

4. Preheat oven to 450°F 20 minutes before you cook the pizza.

5. Bake the pizza for 8 minutes to cook the crust.

6. Top the pizza with the cheese mixture and bake for another 6 to 8 minutes, or until the cheese is melted.

Arugula Cucumber Mint Salad

SERVES 4 TO 6

This refreshing salad is full of fresh flavors, from the crispness of cucumber to the coolness of mint.

⅓ CUP EXTRA-VIRGIN OLIVE OIL

2 TABLESPOONS CHOPPED FRESH MINT

2 TABLESPOONS RED WINE VINEGAR

SALT AND FRESHLY GROUND PEPPER

4 CUPS FRESH ARUGULA

1 SMALL SEEDLESS CUCUMBER, DICED

4 SMALL RADISHES, SLICED THIN

¼ CUP CRUMBLED FETA CHEESE

1. Whisk together the olive oil, mint, and vinegar in a bowl. Season with salt and pepper.

2. Place the arugula in a salad bowl and add the cucumber and radishes. Toss the salad with the dressing to coat.

3. Sprinkle the salad with the feta cheese to serve.

Steamed Mussels in Garlic Wine Broth

SERVES 4

Mussels are incredibly easy to make and they have a lot of unique flavor. In this recipe they pair perfectly with a garlic wine broth.

4 POUNDS LIVE MUSSELS

2 CUPS DRY WHITE WINE

2 MEDIUM SHALLOTS, SLICED

1 TABLESPOON MINCED GARLIC

½ TEASPOON SALT

6 TABLESPOONS BUTTER, CUT INTO PIECES

2 TABLESPOONS CHOPPED FRESH PARSLEY

1 TABLESPOON CHOPPED FRESH BASIL

1 TABLESPOON CHOPPED FRESH CHIVES

1. Rinse the mussels in cool water and scrub them well. Discard any dead mussels and cut the beards from the rest.

2. In a stockpot over medium heat, combine the wine, shallots, garlic. Stir together and simmer the mixture for 5 minutes.

3. Add the mussels, cover, and increase the heat to high. Cook for 5 minutes, or until the mussels have opened. Discard any that do not open.

4. Stir in the butter and herbs and remove the stockpot from the heat.

5. Spoon the mussels and broth into bowls to serve.

Stuffed Bell Peppers

SERVES 4

These stuffed bell peppers get a Mediterranean twist from garlic, feta cheese, and couscous.

4 LARGE RED BELL PEPPERS

ONE 15-OUNCE CAN CANNELLINI BEANS, DRAINED AND RINSED

1 CUP CRUMBLED FETA CHEESE

½ CUP DRY COUSCOUS

1 TEASPOON MINCED GARLIC

1 TEASPOON DRIED OREGANO

SALT AND FRESHLY GROUND PEPPER

¼ CUP SLICED SCALLIONS

1. Slice off the tops of the peppers and remove the ribs and seeds. Discard the stems and chop the tops of the peppers.

2. Put the chopped pepper into a medium bowl. Stir in the beans, feta, couscous, garlic, and oregano. Season with salt and pepper.

3. Spoon the mixture into the peppers and place them in a slow cooker.

4. Cover and cook on high heat for 4 hours.

5. Garnish with sliced scallions to serve.

Hearty Beef
and Sweet Potato Stew

SERVES 4

*If you are looking for a hot and hearty recipe to fill you up, look no further than
this beef and sweet potato stew.*

½ CUP CHOPPED ONION

3 CUPS CHOPPED SWEET POTATO

1¼ POUNDS BEEF STEW MEAT

1½ CUPS BEEF BROTH

1 TABLESPOON MINCED GARLIC

1 TEASPOON GROUND CUMIN

½ TEASPOON GROUND CINNAMON

PINCH OF CAYENNE PEPPER

SALT AND FRESHLY GROUND PEPPER

ONE 14.5-OUNCE CAN DICED TOMATOES

½ CUP DRIED APRICOTS, QUARTERED

1. Combine the onions and sweet potatoes in a 4-quart slow cooker. Stir
in the beef.

2. In a medium bowl, whisk together the broth, garlic, and spices. Season
with salt and pepper. Pour the mixture into the slow cooker.

3. Cover and cook on low heat for 7 to 8 hours.

4. Stir in the diced tomatoes and apricots to serve.

Pan-Seared Scallops with Steamed Veggies

SERVES 4

Scallops are an excellent source of lean protein, not to mention flavor. You don't want any heavy sauces or spices to cover up the natural flavor of these beauties.

2 CUPS BROCCOLI FLORETS

2 CUPS CAULIFLOWER FLORETS

1 CUP BABY CARROTS

2 TABLESPOONS EXTRA-VIRGIN OLIVE OIL

1½ POUNDS LARGE SCALLOPS

SALT AND FRESHLY GROUND PEPPER

1. Place a steamer tray in a large saucepan and fill the pan with 1 to 2 inches of water. Add the vegetables to the pan and cover.

2. Bring the water to a boil and steam the vegetables for 6 to 8 minutes, or until tender. Drain and set aside, covered to keep warm.

3. Heat the oil in a heavy skillet over medium-high heat.

4. Season the scallops with salt and pepper and add them to the skillet.

5. Cook the scallops for 3 minutes on each side, or until cooked through. Serve hot with the vegetables.

Lemon Caper Chicken

SERVES 4

Lemon and capers are a classic Mediterranean combination, and they've never tasted better than in this dish.

FOUR 4-OUNCE SKINLESS CHICKEN BREAST HALVES

SALT AND FRESHLY GROUND PEPPER

1 TABLESPOON EXTRA-VIRGIN OLIVE OIL

⅓ CUP DRY SHERRY

3 TABLESPOONS FRESH LEMON JUICE

2 TABLESPOONS CAPERS

1 TABLESPOON CHOPPED FRESH PARSLEY

1. Season the chicken with salt and pepper.

2. Heat the oil in a skillet over medium-high heat. Add the chicken and cook for 4 to 6 minutes on each side, or until cooked through.

3. Remove the chicken to a plate and cover to keep warm.

4. Whisk together the sherry, lemon juice, and capers in the skillet. Cook until the liquid is reduced to about ¼ cup.

5. Stir in the parsley, and season with salt and pepper.

6. Serve the chicken hot with the caper sauce spooned over it.

Stuffed Portobello Mushroom Caps

If you are looking for a satisfying vegetarian meal, these stuffed mushrooms are sure to do the trick.

FOR THE MARINADE:

6 LARGE PORTOBELLO MUSHROOMS

1 CUP EXTRA-VIRGIN OLIVE OIL

½ CUP BALSAMIC VINEGAR

⅓ CUP SOY SAUCE

1 TABLESPOON MINCED GARLIC

1 TABLESPOON CHOPPED FRESH THYME

SALT AND FRESHLY GROUND PEPPER

FOR THE FILLING:

ONE 10-OUNCE BAG FROZEN SPINACH

1 POUND BUTTON MUSHROOMS

2 TABLESPOONS EXTRA-VIRGIN OLIVE OIL

1 CUP CHOPPED ONION

1 TABLESPOON MINCED GARLIC

SALT AND FRESHLY GROUND PEPPER

½ CUP GRATED PARMESAN CHEESE

¼ CUP PLAIN BREAD CRUMBS

1 CUP CRUMBLED FETA CHEESE

To make the marinade:

1. Clean the mushrooms and remove the stems. Chop the stems and place them in a bowl; set aside.

2. Whisk together oil, vinegar, soy sauce, garlic, and thyme in a bowl and season with salt and pepper.

3. Place the mushroom caps in a glass baking dish and pour the marinade over them. Cover and chill for 4 hours, turning occasionally.

To make the filling:

1. Follow the package directions to cook the spinach. Drain the spinach, allow it to cool, and then squeeze out as much water as you can.

2. Place the button mushrooms in a food processor and add the chopped mushroom stems. Pulse until finely chopped.

3. Transfer the mushrooms to a bowl.

4. Heat the oil in a heavy skillet over medium-high heat. Add the onion and garlic and cook for 4 minutes, stirring.

5. Stir in the chopped mushrooms and season with salt and pepper. Cook until the liquid evaporates, about 6 to 8 minutes.

6. Cool the mushroom mixture to room temperature.

7. Preheat the oven to 400°F.

8. Stir the cooked spinach into the cooked mushroom mixture along with 1/4 cup of Parmesan cheese and the bread crumbs.

9. Stir the mixture well, then toss in the feta cheese. Cover and let stand.

10. Remove the portobello mushrooms from the refrigerator and place them on a baking sheet.

11. Roast the mushroom caps for 15 minutes, then remove them from the oven and spoon the filling into the caps.

12. Sprinkle the filling with the remaining 1/4 cup of Parmesan and bake for 12 to 15 minutes, or until heated through. Serve hot.

Baked Halibut
with Mango Salsa

SERVES 4

This recipe is quick and easy to prepare, but it certainly doesn't lack flavor—the mango salsa sees to that.

FOUR 4- TO 6-OUNCE HALIBUT FILLETS
1 TABLESPOON EXTRA-VIRGIN OLIVE OIL
SALT AND FRESHLY GROUND PEPPER
1 MANGO, PITTED AND CHOPPED
1 NAVEL ORANGE, PEELED AND CHOPPED
3 TABLESPOONS CHOPPED FRESH CILANTRO
1 TABLESPOON MINCED RED ONION
1 TABLESPOON FRESH LEMON JUICE
PINCH OF SALT
PINCH OF FRESHLY GROUND PEPPER

1. Preheat the oven to 350°F.

2. Brush the fish with olive oil and season with salt and pepper. Arrange the fish on a baking sheet.

3. Bake the fish for 12 to 15 minutes, or until it flakes easily with a fork.

4. Meanwhile, combine the remaining ingredients in a bowl. Stir well.

5. Serve the fish hot, topped with the mango salsa.

Strawberry Banana Tart

SERVES 8

There is no reason to feel guilty about this tart, because it is made with fresh fruit and uses whole-wheat flour.

FOR THE CRUST:

1 CUP UNBLEACHED FLOUR

½ CUP WHOLE-WHEAT FLOUR

PINCH OF SALT

¼ CUP EXTRA-VIRGIN OLIVE OIL

¼ CUP CANOLA OIL

2 TABLESPOONS PLAIN NONFAT GREEK YOGURT

1 TEASPOON HONEY

FOR THE FILLING:

¼ CUP SUGAR

¼ CUP PACKED BROWN SUGAR

1 TABLESPOON WHOLE-WHEAT FLOUR

1 TEASPOON GROUND CINNAMON

2 CUPS SLICED STRAWBERRIES

2 BANANAS, SLICED

To make the crust:

1. Preheat the oven to 425°F.

2. Combine the flours and salt in a mixing bowl.

3. In a separate bowl, whisk together the oils, yogurt, and honey. Add the wet ingredients to the dry ingredients and stir until it forms a crumbly mixture.

4. Press the mixture into a tart pan, patting it firmly into the bottom and sides.

continued ▶

To make the filling:

1. Combine the sugars, flour, and cinnamon in a bowl. Add the strawberries and bananas and toss to coat.

2. Spoon the mixture into the tart crust and bake for 45 minutes, or until hot and bubbling.

3. Allow the tart to cool to room temperature before serving.

Spiced Pecans

MAKES 4 CUPS

Sweet and crunchy, with just the right blend of spices, these pecans are a great snack and dessert.

½ CUP SUGAR

1 TEASPOON SALT

1 TEASPOON GROUND CINNAMON

¼ TEASPOON GROUND NUTMEG

⅛ TEASPOON GROUND CLOVES

2 EGG WHITES

4 CUPS WHOLE PECANS

1. Preheat the oven to 300°F.

2. Line two baking sheets with parchment paper.

3. Combine the sugar, salt, cinnamon, nutmeg, and cloves in a small bowl.

4. Whisk the egg whites in a mixing bowl until frothy. Add the spice mixture and whisk until well combined.

5. Add the pecans and stir to coat.

6. Spread the pecans on the baking sheets and bake for 15 minutes.

7. Reduce oven temperature to 250°F and bake for another 10 minutes. Cool the pecans before serving.

Maple Grilled Peaches

SERVES 4

At first glance, you may be skeptical about this recipe. Once you try it, however, you will wonder why you haven't been grilling every peach you eat.

COOKING SPRAY
4 PEACHES, PITTED AND HALVED
1 TABLESPOON CANOLA OIL
¼ CUP MAPLE SYRUP
¼ TEASPOON GROUND CINNAMON

1. Preheat a stovetop grill pan over medium-high heat and lightly grease it with cooking spray.

2. Brush the peaches with ½ tablespoon of canola oil and set them cut-side down on the grill pan.

3. Whisk together the maple syrup and cinnamon with the remaining ½ tablespoon of canola oil. Brush the mixture over the peaches.

4. Grill the peaches for 2 to 4 minutes on each side, brushing occasionally with the maple glaze, until tender. Serve warm.

Blueberry Lime Sorbet

SERVES 6 TO 8

Fresh blueberries and a hint of lime give this sorbet its light and fruity flavor.

4 CUPS FROZEN BLUEBERRIES

¼ CUP SUGAR

¼ CUP HONEY

2 TABLESPOONS FRESH LIME JUICE

1 TABLESPOON LIME ZEST

1. Combine all the ingredients in a mixing bowl and stir well. Mash the ingredients with a potato masher to crush the berries.

2. Transfer the mixture to a blender and blend until smooth.

3. Put the mixture through a sieve and discard the solids.

4. Chill the sorbet for 1 hour, then pour the sorbet into an ice cream maker and freeze according to the manufacturer's directions.

Cranberry Almond Biscotti

SERVES 12

If you aren't a fan of overly sweet desserts, these tart, crunchy biscotti might be just what you are looking for.

1¼ CUPS WHOLE-WHEAT FLOUR

⅓ CUP SUGAR

1 TEASPOON BAKING POWDER

PINCH OF SALT

½ CUP CHOPPED ALMONDS

¼ CUP DRIED CRANBERRIES

2 EGGS

1 TEASPOON ALMOND EXTRACT

1 TEASPOON SKIM MILK

1. Preheat the oven to 350°F.

2. Line a rimmed baking sheet with parchment.

3. Whisk together the flour, sugar, baking powder, and salt in a mixing bowl. Fold in the almonds and cranberries.

4. In another bowl, beat together the eggs, almond extract, and skim milk.

5. Add the wet ingredients to the dry, stirring until just combined.

6. Turn the dough out onto a floured surface and form it into a rectangular loaf.

7. Place the loaf on the baking sheet and bake for 25 minutes, or until it rises. Cool the loaf on a wire rack for 1 hour.

8. Reduce oven temperature to 300°F.

9. Move the loaf to a cutting board and slice it into ¼-inch-thick slices. Arrange the slices on the baking sheet.

10. Bake the slices for 15 minutes; then flip and bake them for another 10 to 15 minutes, or until they are crisp and lightly browned. Cool the biscotti completely before serving.

Apple Cinnamon Scones

SERVES 8

These scones are everything you love about these classic flavors, wrapped in a fluffy pastry.

1 CUP WHOLE-WHEAT FLOUR
1 CUP UNBLEACHED FLOUR
¼ CUP SUGAR
2 TEASPOONS BAKING POWDER
1 TEASPOON GROUND CINNAMON
½ TEASPOON BAKING SODA
¼ TEASPOON GROUND NUTMEG
PINCH OF SALT
¼ CUP COCONUT OIL
1 CUP GRATED APPLE
½ CUP PLAIN NONFAT GREEK YOGURT
1 EGG
1 TEASPOON VANILLA EXTRACT

1. Preheat the oven to 425°F.

2. Line a baking sheet with parchment paper.

3. Combine the dry ingredients in a mixing bowl and blend well. Whisk in the coconut oil and stir until well combined.

4. Add the grated apple, yogurt, egg, and vanilla extract. Stir until just blended.

5. Turn the dough out onto a floured surface and knead several times. Pat the dough into a circle about ¾ inch thick.

6. Use a sharp knife to cut the circle into 8 triangles, then place them on the baking sheet. Bake for 15 to 18 minutes, or until golden brown.

7. Cool the scones for 10 minutes before serving.

Chocolate Bread Pudding

SERVES 8

This pudding is a dream come true—tender and creamy with just the right amount of chocolate flavor.

FOR THE CUSTARD:

COOKING SPRAY

4 EGGS

4 EGG WHITES

1 CUP SKIM MILK

½ CUP SUGAR

1 TABLESPOON VANILLA EXTRACT

½ TEASPOON GROUND CINNAMON

FOR THE FILLING:

4 CUPS WHOLE-GRAIN BREAD, CUBED

2 CUPS PITTED CHERRIES

½ CUP MINI CHOCOLATE CHIPS

¼ CUP CHOPPED TOASTED ALMONDS

To make the custard:

1. Preheat the oven to 375°F.

2. Grease a 2-quart casserole dish with cooking spray.

3. To prepare the custard, whisk together the eggs, egg whites, and milk in a bowl. Whisk in the sugar, vanilla, and cinnamon until smooth.

To make the filling:

1. Toss together the cubed bread, cherries, and chocolate chips in a bowl.

2. Fold the custard into the bread mixture and transfer it to the casserole dish, pressing down to compact the mixture. Cover it with foil.

3. Bake the pudding for 40 to 45 minutes, or until the custard has set. Remove the foil and sprinkle the pudding with chopped almonds.

4. Bake the pudding for another 15 to 20 minutes, or until it is puffy and golden. Cool the pudding for 15 minutes before serving.

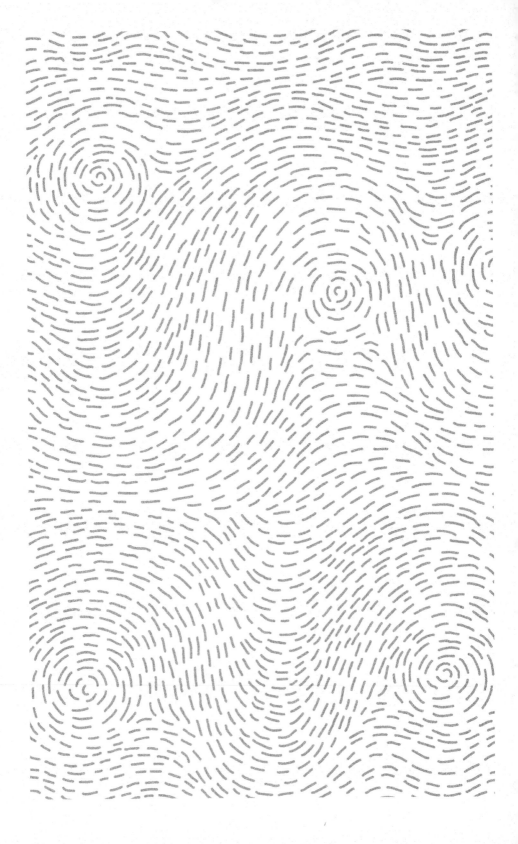

CHAPTER FIVE

Week Three

The Mediterranean diet is a centuries-old tradition that contributes to good health, provides a sense of well-being and pleasure, and forms a vital part of the cultural heritage of these regions. These same practices can be adopted into our homes to enhance our well-being and to reduce our overall risk of heart disease and other chronic disease states.

—Cleveland Clinic Online, "Ask the Dietician: Mediterranean Diet"

WEEK THREE MEAL PLAN

Day One

Breakfast: Egg and Vegetable Breakfast Scramble
Lunch: Tomato Basil Pasta Salad
Dinner: Easy Vegetable Lasagna
Snacks: 1 cup sliced celery; 1 small orange
Dessert: Cinnamon Raisin Scones

Daily Tip: Suffering from foot or joint pain? It could be your sneakers. Wearing old shoes can induce knee pain, so don't skimp when buying your next pair.

Day Two

Breakfast: Whole-Grain Blueberry Muffins
Lunch: Roast Beef Pita Pockets
Dinner: Pork Chops with Roasted Red Peppers
Snacks: 1 sliced kiwi; 3 dark chocolate squares
Dessert: Walnut Mango Smoothie

Daily Tip: If you don't have a lot of time to work out during the week, up the intensity of your workouts. Studies show that shorter-duration, high-intensity activity is just as or more beneficial than prolonged moderate-intensity exercise.

Day Three

Breakfast: Apple Cinnamon Oatmeal
Lunch: Creamy Carrot and Ginger Soup
Dinner: Fettuccine with Parmesan Garlic Sauce
Snacks: 2 tablespoons toasted chickpeas; 14 grapes
Dessert: Kiwi Blueberry Tart

Daily Tip: Consider supplementing your diet with a daily probiotic. Probiotics contain good bacteria that help promote healthy digestion.

Day Four

Breakfast: Zucchini Parmesan Frittata
Lunch: Greek-Style Pasta Salad
Dinner: Grilled Tuna Steaks
Snacks: 4 whole-grain crackers; 1 cup unsweetened applesauce
Dessert: Chocolate Coconut Truffles

Daily Tip: When you go outside, don't forget to protect yourself from the sun. Put on a light sunscreen or a brimmed hat. Avoiding harsh sunlight can help keep your skin looking younger.

Day Five

Breakfast: Blueberry Lemon Pancakes
Lunch: Roasted Tomato Basil Bisque
Dinner: Lemon Herb-Baked Fish
Snacks: 15 whole almonds; 1 hard-boiled egg
Dessert: Whipped Chocolate Mousse

Daily Tip: Go for a walk! If you find yourself feeling tired or run down during the day, you may be craving a nap. What is sure to wake you up, however, is a quick walk.

Day Six

Breakfast: Coconut Raisin Granola
Lunch: Herbed Turkey Meatballs with Pasta
Dinner: Pasta Fagioli
Snacks: 1 cup tomato soup; 1 peach
Dessert: Cherry Walnut Bread Pudding

Daily Tip: Smoking adds to the appearance of wrinkles and fine lines (not to mention the damage it does to your lungs). Quit smoking to add years to your life and take years off your appearance.

Day Seven

Breakfast: Pumpkin Corn Muffins
Lunch: Homemade Falafel Balls
Dinner: Garlic Shrimp and Feta Pasta
Snacks: ¼ cup whole-grain granola; 1 cup chopped watermelon
Dessert: Strawberry Banana Parfaits

Daily Tip: When engaging in exercise, be sure to warm up and cool down properly. This includes stretching.

Note: The snacks included in this meal plan are simple snacks you can purchase from the grocery store that need little to no preparation. For more information regarding the nutritional content of these snacks, refer to Appendix A.

ADDITIONAL TIPS FOR WEEK THREE:

- If you are engaging in a strength-training regimen, focus on your form rather than the size of the plates on the dumbbell. When you lift slowly and properly, your muscles get a better workout than if you rush through.
- Don't stress! Set reasonable limits for yourself at work and at home. Understand your own limits and don't push yourself beyond what you are capable of. There is no harm in challenging yourself, but expecting too much of yourself or others can lead to an unhealthful amount of stress.
- Include bananas in your diet. Bananas are packed with potassium, and they have been shown to help reduce sodium.

WEEK THREE SHOPPING LIST

To prepare your meals for this week, purchase the following items in the quantities indicated:

Pantry Items

- Basil, dried
- Cinnamon, ground
- Cumin, ground
- Oregano, dried
- Pepper
- Pumpkin pie spice
- Salt
- Thyme, dried
- Canola oil
- Coconut oil
- Cooking spray
- Olive oil, extra-virgin
- Walnut oil
- Coconut extract
- Vanilla extract
- Baking powder
- Baking soda
- Cocoa powder, unsweetened
- Vinegar, apple cider
- Vinegar, balsamic
- Vinegar, red wine
- Honey
- Maple syrup
- Coconut butter
- Garlic
- Ginger, fresh

Produce

- Basil (2 bunches)
- Chives (1 bunch)
- Cilantro (1 bunch)
- Parsley (1 bunch)
- Apple (1 small)
- Bananas (2 medium)
- Blueberries (4 cups)
- Cherries, pitted (2 cups)
- Kiwi (2)
- Lemons (5)
- Strawberries (1 cup)
- Bell peppers, green (1)
- Bell peppers, red (5)
- Carrots (2 bags)
- Cucumber (1 small)
- Lettuce, shredded (2 cups)
- Onions (3 medium)
- Onions, red (2 medium)
- Potato, yellow (1 medium)
- Scallion (1 small)
- Squash, summer (1 medium)
- Tomatoes (12 medium)
- Zucchini (3 medium)
- White mushrooms (1 cup)

Protein

- Beef, deli roast (½ pound)
- Haddock fillets (four, 4 to 6 ounces)
- Pork chops, large (4)
- Shrimp, raw (1 pound)
- Tuna steaks (four, 1-inch thick)
- Turkey, lean ground (1 pound)

Dairy

- Cream, heavy (2 cups)
- Milk, skim (3¼ cups)
- Feta cheese, crumbled (2½ cups)
- Goat cheese, crumbled (1¾ cups)
- Parmesan cheese, grated (¾ cup)
- Yogurt, plain nonfat Greek (1½ cups)
- Yogurt, vanilla nonfat Greek (2 cups)

Dry Foods

- Baking mix (1 cup)
- Flour, bulgur (¼ cup)
- Flour, unbleached (2 cups)
- Flour, whole-wheat (3⅔ cups)
- Sugar (1¼ cups)
- Sugar, brown (1¼ cups)
- Bread crumbs, plain (1 cup)
- Coconut, unsweetened flaked (¾ cup)
- Cornmeal, yellow (1 cup)
- Oats, old-fashioned (2 cups)
- Oats, rolled (1 cup)
- Oats, steel-cut (1 cup)
- Fettuccine, whole-wheat (8 ounces)
- Lasagna noodles, whole-wheat (1 pound)
- Linguine, whole-wheat (8 ounces)
- Macaroni, whole-wheat (20 ounces)
- Penne, whole-wheat (16 ounces)
- Beans, white cannellini (one 15-ounce can)
- Chickpeas, dried (1 cup)
- Dates, pitted (⅔ cup)
- Raisins (1½ cups)
- Almonds, slivered (⅓ cup)
- Granola, whole-grain (½ cup)
- Walnuts, chopped (1¼ cups)

Refrigerated and Frozen Foods

- Eggs (30)
- Mango chunks, frozen (2 cups)

Other

- Bread, whole-grain (4 cups cubed)
- Pita pockets, whole-wheat (4)
- Applesauce, unsweetened (2 cups)
- Black olives, sliced (½ cup)
- Capers (2 tablespoons)
- Chocolate, bittersweet (7 ounces)
- Marinara sauce (6 cups)
- Pumpkin purée (¾ cup)
- Red bell pepper, roasted (⅓ cup)
- Tomatoes, diced (three 15-ounce cans)
- Tomatoes, Italian-style (one 16-ounce can)
- Vinegar, sherry (¼ cup)
- White wine, dry (1 cup)
- Broth, chicken (4 cups)
- Broth, vegetable (4 cups)

PLAN-AHEAD PREPARATIONS

There are several things you can prepare ahead of time and use throughout the week to make your life easier.

1. **Sliced black olives:** You will use these in several recipes. If you prefer not to buy pre-sliced olives, purchase them whole and slice them yourself using a small, sharp knife.
2. **Sliced vegetables:** You can never have enough sliced vegetables on hand. This week you will use sliced vegetables in various salads and entrées. You can use whatever vegetables you like, but some recommendations include zucchini, broccoli, carrots, mushrooms, tomatoes, and summer squash.
3. **Chopped greens:** Again, chopped greens are a staple in the Mediterranean diet, and this week you will use them in smoothies as well as salads. Chop a bag's worth of kale, romaine lettuce, and whatever other greens you enjoy in your salad to have on hand.
4. **Fresh lemon juice:** Lemon juice will be used in several recipes this week. Juice several lemons at a time and store the juice in an airtight container in the fridge.

WEEK THREE RECIPES

Breakfast Recipes

EGG AND VEGETABLE BREAKFAST SCRAMBLE

WHOLE-GRAIN BLUEBERRY MUFFINS

APPLE CINNAMON OATMEAL

ZUCCHINI PARMESAN FRITTATA

BLUEBERRY LEMON PANCAKES

COCONUT RAISIN GRANOLA

PUMPKIN CORN MUFFINS

Lunch Recipes

TOMATO BASIL PASTA SALAD

ROAST BEEF PITA POCKETS

CREAMY CARROT AND GINGER SOUP

GREEK-STYLE PASTA SALAD

ROASTED TOMATO BASIL BISQUE

HERBED TURKEY MEATBALLS WITH PASTA

HOMEMADE FALAFEL BALLS

Dinner Recipes

EASY VEGETABLE LASAGNA

PORK CHOPS WITH ROASTED RED PEPPERS

FETTUCCINE WITH PARMESAN GARLIC SAUCE

GRILLED TUNA STEAKS

LEMON HERB-BAKED FISH

PASTA FAGIOLI

GARLIC SHRIMP AND FETA PASTA

Dessert Recipes

CINNAMON RAISIN SCONES

WALNUT MANGO SMOOTHIE

KIWI BLUEBERRY TART

CHOCOLATE COCONUT TRUFFLES

WHIPPED CHOCOLATE MOUSSE

CHERRY WALNUT BREAD PUDDING

STRAWBERRY BANANA PARFAITS

Egg and Vegetable Breakfast Scramble

SERVES 2

This egg and vegetable scramble is easy to make for a crowd—simply multiply the recipe by two (or even three) to suit your needs.

3 EGGS

1 TABLESPOON SKIM MILK

2 TEASPOONS EXTRA-VIRGIN OLIVE OIL

1 TEASPOON MINCED GARLIC

½ SMALL RED ONION, CHOPPED

½ SMALL GREEN BELL PEPPER, SEEDED AND CHOPPED

½ CUP CHOPPED WHITE MUSHROOMS

1 SCALLION, SLICED

SALT AND FRESHLY GROUND PEPPER

1. Whisk together the eggs and skim milk in a small bowl and set aside.

2. Heat the olive oil in a skillet over medium-high heat. Add the garlic and cook for 1 minute.

3. Stir in the onion, bell pepper, and mushrooms, and cook for 4 to 5 minutes, or until tender.

4. Remove the vegetables from the skillet and put them in a bowl. Pour the egg mixture into the hot skillet.

5. Tilt the skillet to spread the egg mixture and cook it for 30 seconds.

6. Use a spatula to stir the eggs slowly as they cook, cooking for 2 to 3 minutes, or until just set.

7. Stir the cooked vegetables back into the skillet and cook until heated through.

8. Toss with the scallion, season with salt and pepper, and serve.

Whole-Grain Blueberry Muffins

MAKES 12 MUFFINS

A healthier option than store-bought muffins, these whole-grain muffins are a great way to start your day.

1 CUP ROLLED OATS

1 CUP WHOLE-WHEAT FLOUR

1 TEASPOON GROUND CINNAMON

1 TEASPOON BAKING SODA

½ TEASPOON SALT

1 CUP UNSWEETENED APPLESAUCE

½ CUP RAW HONEY

2 EGGS

1 TEASPOON VANILLA EXTRACT

1 CUP FRESH BLUEBERRIES

1. Preheat the oven to 325°F.

2. Combine the oats, flour, cinnamon, baking soda, and salt in a medium mixing bowl and stir well.

3. In a separate mixing bowl, beat the applesauce, honey, eggs, and vanilla extract until smooth.

4. Add the dry ingredients to the wet ingredients in small batches, stirring until smooth after each addition.

5. Fold in the fresh blueberries and stir until just combined.

6. Line a muffin tin with paper liners and fill each cup about two-thirds full with batter.

7. Bake for 20 to 25 minutes, or until a knife inserted in the center comes out clean.

8. Cool the muffins in the pan for 5 minutes; then turn them out onto a wire cooling rack to cool completely before serving.

Apple Cinnamon Oatmeal

SERVES 4

If you are an oatmeal lover, you are sure to enjoy this tasty hot breakfast. And if you don't normally enjoy oatmeal, this recipe might make you change your mind.

2 CUPS WATER

1 CUP STEEL-CUT OATS

¼ CUP GRATED APPLE

½ TEASPOON GROUND CINNAMON

PINCH OF SALT

1 TABLESPOON MAPLE SYRUP

1. Whisk together the water and steel-cut oats in a small saucepan over medium heat.

2. Add the apple, cinnamon, and salt.

3. Bring to a boil, then reduce heat and simmer on low, uncovered, for about 20 minutes.

4. Spoon the oatmeal into bowls and top with a drizzle of maple syrup to serve.

Zucchini Parmesan Frittata

SERVES 6

This frittata is unique in terms of flavor but familiar enough that even the pickiest of eaters will love it.

1 TABLESPOON EXTRA-VIRGIN OLIVE OIL

2 CUPS CHOPPED ZUCCHINI

½ TEASPOON DRIED BASIL

½ TEASPOON DRIED OREGANO

½ TEASPOON DRIED THYME

SALT AND FRESHLY GROUND PEPPER

½ CUP CRUMBLED FETA CHEESE

¼ CUP GRATED PARMESAN CHEESE

8 EGGS, BEATEN

1. Preheat the broiler to high heat.

2. Heat the olive oil in an ovenproof skillet over medium heat. Add the zucchini and toss to coat with oil.

3. Cook the zucchini for 2 minutes, then stir in the dried spices and season with salt and pepper. Cook for 6 to 7 minutes more, or until tender.

4. Reduce the heat to low and sprinkle the two cheeses over the zucchini. Pour in the beaten eggs and stir gently.

5. Cover the skillet and cook on low for 15 minutes, or until the frittata is almost set.

6. Uncover the skillet and place it under the broiler for 2 minutes, until browned. Let it sit for 5 minutes before serving.

Blueberry Lemon Pancakes

SERVES 3

There is nothing better than a stack of blueberry pancakes—except maybe a stack of these blueberry lemon pancakes.

1 CUP SKIM MILK

1 TABLESPOON APPLE CIDER VINEGAR

1 CUP WHOLE-WHEAT FLOUR

½ TEASPOON BAKING POWDER

¼ TEASPOON BAKING SODA

1 EGG

2 TABLESPOONS CANOLA OIL

2 TABLESPOONS FRESH LEMON JUICE

1 TABLESPOON LEMON ZEST

1 TABLESPOON HONEY

1 CUP FRESH BLUEBERRIES

1. Whisk together the milk and vinegar in a small bowl. Set aside.

2. In another bowl, stir together the flour, baking powder, and baking soda.

3. Beat the egg with the canola oil, lemon juice, lemon zest, and honey in a medium mixing bowl. Add the milk mixture and whisk until smooth.

4. Whisk in the dry ingredients in small batches, stirring until smooth between each addition.

5. Heat a nonstick skillet over medium-high heat. Spoon the batter onto the hot skillet in heaping tablespoonfuls.

6. Drop a few blueberries into each pancake.

7. Let the pancakes cook until the batter begins to bubble on the surface, 1 to 2 minutes. Carefully flip the pancakes and cook for 1 to 2 minutes more, or until the underside is lightly browned.

8. Transfer the cooked pancakes to a plate and repeat with the remaining batter.

Coconut Raisin Granola

SERVES 6

There is nothing like a bowl of homemade granola for breakfast in the morning. Crunchy and flavorful, it will keep you satisfied all morning long.

2 CUPS OLD-FASHIONED OATS

½ CUP UNSWEETENED FLAKED COCONUT

⅓ CUP SLIVERED ALMONDS

¼ CUP CHOPPED WALNUTS

1 TEASPOON GROUND CINNAMON

PINCH OF SALT

3 TABLESPOONS CANOLA OIL

¼ CUP HONEY

¼ CUP PACKED BROWN SUGAR

1 TEASPOON COCONUT EXTRACT

½ CUP RAISINS

1. Preheat the oven to 375°F.

2. Line a rimmed baking sheet with parchment paper.

3. Combine the old-fashioned oats, coconut, almonds, and walnuts in a large mixing bowl with the cinnamon and salt. Toss well.

4. In a small bowl, whisk together the canola oil, honey, brown sugar, and coconut extract.

5. Pour the canola oil mixture over the oat mixture and mix well by hand until the oats are coated. Spread the oat mixture out on the prepared baking sheet.

6. Bake for 10 minutes, then turn the granola with a spatula and bake 5 to 10 minutes more, or until just browned.

7. Transfer the mixture to a large bowl to cool and stir in the raisins. Store in an airtight container for up to 5 days.

Pumpkin Corn Muffins

MAKES 12 MUFFINS

You may not be used to having corn muffins for breakfast, but these muffins are sure to turn you into a believer.

3 EGGS

½ CUP EXTRA-VIRGIN OLIVE OIL

¾ CUP PUMPKIN PURÉE

¾ CUP PACKED BROWN SUGAR

1 TEASPOON VANILLA EXTRACT

1½ TEASPOONS PUMPKIN PIE SPICE

1 CUP YELLOW CORNMEAL

1 CUP BAKING MIX

1 TEASPOON BAKING POWDER

¼ TEASPOON SALT

1. Preheat the oven to 350°F.

2. Line a muffin pan with paper liners.

3. Beat the eggs in a large mixing bowl until frothy, then beat in the oil. Add the pumpkin purée and beat until smooth.

4. Whisk the brown sugar, vanilla extract, and pumpkin pie spice into the egg mixture until smooth.

5. In a separate bowl, whisk together the cornmeal, baking mix, baking powder, and salt. Whisk the mixture into the wet ingredients in small batches until smooth and well combined.

6. Drop the batter into the prepared muffin pan, filling each cup about two-thirds full. Bake for 20 minutes, or until a knife inserted in the center comes out clean.

7. Cool the muffins in the pan for 5 minutes; then turn the muffins out onto wire racks to cool completely before serving.

Lunch Recipes

Tomato Basil Pasta Salad

SERVES 6 TO 8

This healthful pasta salad is a tasty twist on traditional pasta salad. Tossed with fresh tomatoes and basil, this is one pasta salad you won't get sick of.

SALT

12 OUNCES WHOLE-WHEAT MACARONI

3½ CUPS CHOPPED TOMATOES

¼ CUP CHOPPED RED ONION

¼ CUP EXTRA-VIRGIN OLIVE OIL

2 TABLESPOONS RED WINE VINEGAR

1 GARLIC CLOVE, MINCED

½ TEASPOON DRIED OREGANO

FRESHLY GROUND PEPPER

1 CUP CHOPPED FRESH BASIL

1. Bring a pot of salted water to a boil and cook the pasta al dente according to the package directions. Drain and set aside.

2. Combine the tomatoes, onion, olive oil, vinegar, garlic, and oregano in a bowl. Season with salt and pepper and toss to coat.

3. Let the mixture sit at room temperature for 30 minutes.

4. Rinse the pasta in cool water and drain. Add it to the tomato mixture and toss to coat the pasta. Stir in the basil.

5. Chill until ready to serve.

Roast Beef Pita Pockets

SERVES 4

These beef pita pockets are quick to throw together and make an excellent option for school lunches or a lunch break at the office.

½ POUND ROAST BEEF, THINLY SLICED AND CUT INTO STRIPS

2 CUPS SHREDDED LETTUCE

1 CUP GRATED CARROT

1 CUP DICED CUCUMBER

½ CUP THINLY SLICED RED ONION

½ CUP CRUMBLED FETA CHEESE

2 TABLESPOONS PLAIN NONFAT GREEK YOGURT

2 TABLESPOONS SKIM MILK

1 TABLESPOON APPLE CIDER VINEGAR

SALT AND FRESHLY GROUND PEPPER

4 WHOLE-WHEAT PITA POCKETS

1. Combine the beef, lettuce, carrot, cucumber, onion, and feta in a bowl and stir well.

2. In a separate bowl, whisk together the Greek yogurt, milk, and vinegar. Season with salt and pepper.

3. Cut about one-fourth off each pita and stuff the remaining pita with the beef mixture. Spoon the dressing on top and serve.

Creamy Carrot and Ginger Soup

SERVES 4

If you want something warm and creamy for lunch, try this carrot and ginger soup. The fresh ginger gives it a unique depth of flavor you are sure to love.

4 CUPS CHICKEN BROTH

1 TABLESPOON MINCED GARLIC

1 CUP CHOPPED ONION

½ TABLESPOON GRATED FRESH GINGER

1 POUND CARROTS, PEELED AND CHOPPED

1 MEDIUM YELLOW POTATO, CHOPPED

SALT AND FRESHLY GROUND PEPPER

2 TABLESPOONS CHOPPED CHIVES, FOR GARNISH

1. Heat ½ cup of broth in a saucepan over medium-high heat. Add the garlic and onion and cook for 5 minutes, or until the onion is tender.

2. Add the ginger, carrots, and potato and stir in the remaining 3½ cups of broth. Season with salt and pepper. Bring to a boil.

3. Reduce the heat and simmer for 25 minutes, or until the carrots are tender.

4. Remove the soup from the heat and purée it using an immersion blender. Serve hot, garnished with the chopped chives.

Greek-Style Pasta Salad

SERVES 2

This Greek pasta salad is studded with sliced olives and capers, and tossed with a vinaigrette dressing and crumbled feta cheese. What could be more Greek than that?

SALT

8 OUNCES WHOLE-WHEAT PENNE

¼ CUP EXTRA-VIRGIN OLIVE OIL

1 TABLESPOON BALSAMIC VINEGAR

1 TABLESPOON MINCED GARLIC

½ TEASPOON DRIED OREGANO

FRESHLY GROUND PEPPER

1 CUP CHOPPED TOMATOES

⅓ CUP ROASTED RED BELL PEPPER, CHOPPED

2 TABLESPOONS CAPERS

¼ CUP SLICED BLACK OLIVES

½ CUP CRUMBLED FETA CHEESE

1. Bring a pot of salted water to a boil and cook the pasta al dente according to the package directions. Drain and set aside.

2. Whisk together the olive oil, vinegar, garlic, and oregano in a small bowl, and season with salt and pepper. Set aside.

3. Combine the tomatoes, bell pepper, capers, and olives in a large bowl. Toss the mixture with the dressing and let it sit for 15 minutes.

4. Stir in the pasta, and toss with feta crumbles. Serve at room temperature, or refrigerate to serve later.

Roasted Tomato Basil Bisque

SERVES 4 TO 6

A tasty twist on traditional tomato soup, this roasted tomato bisque tastes like nothing you've ever eaten from a can. After trying this recipe you may find yourself avoiding the soup aisle.

2½ POUNDS TOMATOES, HALVED

1 MEDIUM ONION, CHOPPED

4 TABLESPOONS EXTRA-VIRGIN OLIVE OIL

SALT AND FRESHLY GROUND PEPPER

1 TABLESPOON MINCED GARLIC

ONE 15-OUNCE CAN DICED TOMATOES

1 CUP CHOPPED FRESH BASIL

4 CUPS VEGETABLE BROTH

1. Preheat the oven to 400°F.

2. Spread the fresh tomatoes on a baking sheet and sprinkle them with the onion. Drizzle the tomatoes with 2 tablespoons of olive oil and season with salt and pepper.

3. Roast the tomatoes and onions for 45 minutes, or until tender.

4. Heat the remaining 2 tablespoons of oil in a stockpot over medium heat. Stir in the garlic and cook for 1 minute.

5. Add the canned tomatoes, basil, and vegetable broth. Stir in the roasted tomatoes and onions. Simmer for 30 minutes.

6. Remove the soup from the heat and purée it using an immersion blender, or in batches in a traditional blender. Season with salt and pepper, and serve hot.

Herbed Turkey Meatballs with Pasta

SERVES 4 TO 6

These turkey meatballs are bursting with flavor; they're the perfect companion to freshly cooked pasta and marinara sauce.

SALT

8 OUNCES WHOLE-WHEAT LINGUINE

1 POUND LEAN GROUND TURKEY

2 TABLESPOONS CHOPPED FRESH BASIL

2 TABLESPOONS CHOPPED FRESH PARSLEY

1 TEASPOON DRIED OREGANO

FRESHLY GROUND PEPPER

2 TABLESPOONS EXTRA-VIRGIN OLIVE OIL

2 CUPS STORE-BOUGHT MARINARA SAUCE

1. Bring a pot of salted water to a boil and cook the pasta al dente according to the package directions. Drain and set aside.

2. Combine the turkey, basil, parsley, and oregano in a mixing bowl and mix well. Season with salt and pepper. Shape the mixture by hand into 2-inch balls.

3. Heat the oil in a skillet over medium-high heat.

4. Add the meatballs and cook until browned, about 5 minutes, turning as needed.

5. Pour in the marinara sauce and bring to a simmer. Cover the skillet and cook until the meatballs are cooked through, about 5 to 10 minutes longer.

6. Add the drained pasta to the skillet and toss to coat with the sauce. Transfer the meatballs and pasta to a large bowl to serve.

Homemade Falafel Balls

MAKES 20 FALAFEL BALLS

If you love falafel, you are definitely going to want to try this recipe. It is as good as anything you could find at your local Mediterranean restaurant.

1 CUP DRIED CHICKPEAS
1 CUP CHOPPED ONIONS
2 TABLESPOONS CHOPPED FRESH PARSLEY
2 TABLESPOONS CHOPPED FRESH CILANTRO
1 TABLESPOON MINCED GARLIC
1 TEASPOON GROUND CUMIN
SALT
1 TEASPOON BAKING POWDER
4 TABLESPOONS BULGUR FLOUR
CANOLA OIL FOR FRYING

1. Cover the chickpeas with water and soak overnight. Drain the chickpeas and rinse them well.

2. Combine the chickpeas and onions in a food processor and pulse to chop. Add the herbs, garlic, and cumin. Season with salt.

3. Process the mixture until well blended but not puréed.

4. Sprinkle the baking powder and flour over the mixture and pulse until it forms a ball.

5. Turn the mixture out into a bowl, cover, and chill for 3 to 4 hours.

6. Shape the chickpea mixture into 20 balls and set them on a plate.

7. Heat the oil to 375°F in a deep skillet. Add the falafel balls and cook until browned, about 2 to 3 minutes on each side.

8. Drain the falafel balls on paper towels to serve.

Easy Vegetable Lasagna

SERVES 8

This vegetable lasagna is a vegetarian-friendly twist on an Italian favorite. It's good for the whole family.

1¾ CUPS CRUMBLED GOAT CHEESE

¼ CUP SLICED BLACK OLIVES

1 TEASPOON DRIED THYME

1 TEASPOON DRIED BASIL

¼ TEASPOON DRIED OREGANO

1 TABLESPOON MINCED GARLIC

SALT AND FRESHLY GROUND PEPPER

4 CUPS STORE-BOUGHT MARINARA SAUCE

1 POUND WHOLE-WHEAT LASAGNA NOODLES, COOKED

1 MEDIUM ZUCCHINI, SLICED

1 MEDIUM SUMMER SQUASH, SLICED

1 RED BELL PEPPER, SEEDED AND SLICED THIN

3 TABLESPOONS GRATED PARMESAN CHEESE

1. Preheat the oven to 375°F.

2. Combine the goat cheese, olives, herbs, and garlic in a bowl. Season with salt and pepper.

3. Lightly grease an 8-by-11-inch glass baking dish. Spread 1 cup of marinara sauce in the bottom.

4. Place a layer of cooked noodles over the sauce and top them with a layer of zucchini, squash, and bell pepper.

5. Spoon tablespoons of the goat cheese mixture over the vegetables, spreading evenly.

6. Repeat this process to create additional layers, ending with cooked pasta and sauce. Top with the Parmesan cheese.

7. Cover the lasagna with foil and bake it for 40 minutes. Remove the foil and bake the lasagna 5 minutes longer, or until the cheese browns.

8. Let the lasagna stand for 10 minutes before serving.

Pork Chops with Roasted Red Peppers

SERVES 4 TO 6

Thick, juicy pork chops cooked with garlic and roasted peppers—is your mouth watering yet?

4 RED BELL PEPPERS
2 TABLESPOONS EXTRA-VIRGIN OLIVE OIL
4 LARGE PORK CHOPS
1 TABLESPOON MINCED GARLIC
1 CUP DRY WHITE WINE
¼ CUP SHERRY VINEGAR
SALT AND FRESHLY GROUND PEPPER

1. Preheat the broiler.

2. Place the peppers on a broiler pan below the broiler. Turning the peppers often, cook until they are charred on all sides, about 5 minutes.

3. Seal the peppers in a plastic bag and let them sit for 15 minutes. Remove the peels, seeds, and ribs from the peppers and chop coarsely.

4. Heat the olive oil in a heavy skillet over high heat. Add the pork chops and cook for 2 minutes on each side, or until browned.

5. Add the garlic to the skillet and cook for 1 minute.

6. Stir in the white wine and cook for 3 minutes, scraping up the browned bits in the skillet.

7. Add the chopped peppers and vinegar, swirling the pan for 2 minutes. Season with salt and pepper.

8. Reduce the heat and cover, cooking until the pork chops are cooked through, 4 to 5 minutes. Serve hot.

Fettuccine with Parmesan Garlic Sauce

SERVES 4

Similar to a classic fettuccine Alfredo, this recipe is one that the whole family is sure to love.

SALT

8 OUNCES WHOLE-WHEAT FETTUCCINE

3 TABLESPOONS EXTRA-VIRGIN OLIVE OIL

1 TABLESPOON MINCED GARLIC

1 CUP PLAIN BREAD CRUMBS

3 TABLESPOONS FRESH LEMON JUICE

FRESHLY GROUND PEPPER

½ CUP CHOPPED FRESH PARSLEY

¼ CUP GRATED PARMESAN CHEESE

1. Bring a pot of salted water to a boil and add the fettuccine. Cook al dente according to the package directions. Drain and set aside.

2. Heat 1½ tablespoons of olive oil in a skillet over medium heat. Add the garlic and cook for 1 minute. Spoon the garlic into a bowl and set aside.

3. Heat the remaining 1½ tablespoons of oil in the skillet and stir in the bread crumbs. Cook, stirring often, until they are golden brown.

4. Transfer the bread crumbs to a plate.

5. Whisk together the lemon juice and garlic in a serving bowl and season with salt and pepper. Add the cooked pasta and toss with the chopped parsley and grated Parmesan cheese.

6. Sprinkle with the bread crumbs to serve.

Grilled Tuna Steaks

SERVES 4

These tuna steaks are incredibly simple to make and are simply delicious. They have to chill overnight, so plan ahead for an easy meal the next night.

4 TUNA STEAKS, ABOUT 1 INCH THICK
1 TABLESPOON MINCED GARLIC
SALT AND FRESHLY GROUND PEPPER
ZEST FROM 1 LEMON
EXTRA-VIRGIN OLIVE OIL FOR DRIZZLING

1. Rub the tuna steaks with garlic and season with salt and pepper.

2. Place the steaks in a shallow dish close together. Sprinkle them with the lemon zest and drizzle with the olive oil.

3. Cover the steaks tightly and chill them overnight.

4. Preheat the grill to high heat.

5. Add the steaks. Cook until the steaks turn beige about one-third of the way up their sides, about 1 minute on each side.

6. Carefully flip the steaks and cook until only a sliver of pink remains in the middle. Serve hot.

Lemon Herb-Baked Fish

SERVES 4

If you are in need of a quick but flavorful meal, try this baked fish. It takes only about five minutes to prepare and fifteen minutes to cook.

COOKING SPRAY

FOUR 4- TO 6-OUNCE HADDOCK FILLETS

SALT AND FRESHLY GROUND PEPPER

1 TEASPOON DRIED OREGANO

½ TEASPOON DRIED THYME

½ TEASPOON DRIED BASIL

1 SMALL LEMON, SLICED THIN

1. Preheat the oven to 350°F.

2. Lightly grease a baking sheet with cooking spray.

3. Season the fish with salt and pepper and place them on the baking sheet.

4. Combine the herbs in a small bowl and sprinkle them over the fish.

5. Cover the fish with the lemon slices and bake for 12 to 15 minutes, or until the fillets flake easily with a fork. Serve hot.

Pasta Fagioli

SERVES 4

Pasta fagioli is traditionally made with pasta and beans. In this recipe, tender whole-wheat pasta is combined with white cannellini beans in a flavorful sauce.

SALT

8 OUNCES WHOLE-WHEAT MACARONI

2½ TABLESPOON EXTRA-VIRGIN OLIVE OIL

1 TEASPOON MINCED GARLIC

ONE 16-OUNCE CAN ITALIAN TOMATOES, DRAINED AND CHOPPED

1 TEASPOON DRIED BASIL

ONE 15-OUNCE CAN WHITE CANNELLINI BEANS, DRAINED AND RINSED

2 TABLESPOONS CHOPPED FRESH PARSLEY

FRESHLY GROUND PEPPER

1. Bring a pot of salted water to a boil and add the macaroni. Cook al dente according to the package directions. Drain and set aside.

2. Heat the oil in a deep skillet over medium heat.

3. Add the garlic and cook for 1 minute.

4. Stir in the tomatoes and cook for 5 minutes more, stirring.

5. Stir the herbs into the tomato mixture and cook for about 15 minutes, or until the tomatoes are tender.

6. Add the beans and cook for 5 minutes, or until heated through.

7. Add the parsley and season with salt and pepper.

8. Stir in the macaroni and cook until heated through. Serve hot.

Garlic Shrimp and Feta Pasta

SERVES 4

This shrimp and feta pasta is perfect for a nice dinner at home.

2 TABLESPOONS EXTRA-VIRGIN OLIVE OIL

1 TEASPOON MINCED GARLIC

1 MEDIUM ONION, DICED

1 TEASPOON DRIED OREGANO

½ TEASPOON DRIED THYME

SALT AND FRESHLY GROUND PEPPER

TWO 15-OUNCE CANS DICED TOMATOES

8 OUNCES WHOLE-WHEAT PENNE

1 POUND RAW SHRIMP, PEELED AND DEVEINED

1 CUP CRUMBLED FETA CHEESE

1. Heat the oil in a deep skillet over medium heat. Add the garlic and cook for 1 minute.

2. Stir in the onion and spices, and season with salt and pepper. Cook for 5 minutes, stirring often.

3. Add the tomatoes and bring to a simmer. Simmer for 20 to 25 minutes, or until the tomatoes are tender.

4. Bring a pot of salted water to a boil and cook the pasta al dente according to the package directions. Drain and set aside.

5. Stir the shrimp into the tomato mixture and cook for 2 to 3 minutes, or until the shrimp begin to curl.

6. Remove the shrimp from the heat; stir in the cooked pasta and crumbled feta. Serve hot.

Cinnamon Raisin Scones

SERVES 8

Scones are not something in the average person's repertoire, but after trying these cinnamon-scented scones, you may find yourself making them quite often.

1 CUP WHOLE-WHEAT FLOUR

1 CUP UNBLEACHED FLOUR

2 TEASPOON BAKING POWDER

2 TEASPOON GROUND CINNAMON

½ TEASPOON BAKING SODA

PINCH OF SALT

¼ CUP SUGAR

¼ CUP COCONUT OIL

1 CUP UNSWEETENED APPLESAUCE

½ CUP PLAIN NONFAT GREEK YOGURT

1 EGG

1 TEASPOON VANILLA EXTRACT

1 CUP RAISINS

1. Preheat the oven to 425°F.

2. Line a baking sheet with parchment paper.

3. Combine the dry ingredients in a mixing bowl and blend well. Whisk in the coconut oil and stir until well combined.

4. Add the applesauce, yogurt, egg, and vanilla extract. Stir until just blended.

5. Fold in the raisins.

6. Turn the dough out onto a floured surface and knead several times. Pat the dough into a circle about ¾-inch thick.

7. Use a sharp knife to cut the circle into 8 triangles; place them on the baking sheet. Bake for 15 to 18 minutes, or until the scones are golden brown.

8. Cool the scones for 10 minutes before serving.

Walnut Mango Smoothie

Mango and walnut pair beautifully in this sweet and simple smoothie.

2 CUPS CHOPPED FROZEN MANGO

1 CUP SKIM MILK

½ CUP PLAIN NONFAT GREEK YOGURT

3 TABLESPOONS CHOPPED WALNUTS

½ TEASPOON WALNUT OIL

1. Combine all the ingredients in a blender and blend until smooth and well combined.

2. Pour the smoothie into two glasses and serve immediately.

Kiwi Blueberry Tart

SERVES 8

Made using whole-wheat flour and topped with fresh kiwi and blueberries, this tart is to die for.

FOR THE CRUST:

1 CUP UNBLEACHED FLOUR

½ CUP WHOLE-WHEAT FLOUR

PINCH OF SALT

¼ CUP EXTRA-VIRGIN OLIVE OIL

¼ CUP CANOLA OIL

2 TABLESPOONS PLAIN NONFAT GREEK YOGURT

1 TEASPOON HONEY

FOR THE FILLING:

¼ CUP SUGAR

¼ CUP PACKED BROWN SUGAR

1 TABLESPOON WHOLE-WHEAT FLOUR

1 TEASPOON GROUND CINNAMON

2 CUPS FRESH BLUEBERRIES

1 CUP SLICED KIWI

To make the crust:

1. Preheat the oven to 425°F.

2. Combine the flours and salt in a mixing bowl.

3. In a separate bowl, whisk together the oils, yogurt, and honey. Add the wet ingredients to the dry ingredients and whisk until it forms a crumbly dough.

4. Press the dough into a tart pan, patting it firmly into the bottom and sides.

To make the filling:

1. Combine the sugars, flour, and cinnamon in a bowl. Add the blueberries and kiwi and toss to coat.

2. Spoon the mixture into the tart crust and bake for 45 minutes, or until hot and bubbling.

3. Allow to cool for 10 minutes then serve warm.

Chocolate Coconut Truffles

MAKES 6

These truffles are simple to put together and made with wholesome ingredients—no guilt necessary!

⅔ CUP PITTED DATES

3 TABLESPOONS UNSWEETENED FLAKED COCONUT

1½ TABLESPOONS COCONUT BUTTER

1 TABLESPOON HONEY

1 TABLESPOON UNSWEETENED COCOA POWDER

1. Combine all the ingredients in a food processor and blend until they start to stick together.

2. Roll the mixture into 6 balls by hand and place on a plate. Chill until firm, about 15 minutes.

Whipped Chocolate Mousse

SERVES 4

Everyone loves a little chocolate mousse. With this recipe, you can whip up a batch at home whenever you like.

2 CUPS UNSWEETENED CANNED COCONUT MILK

4 LARGE EGG YOLKS

¼ CUP SUGAR

PINCH OF SALT

1 TEASPOON VANILLA EXTRACT

7 OUNCES CHOPPED BITTERSWEET CHOCOLATE

1. Heat ¾ cup of the coconut milk in a saucepan until steaming; do not let it boil.

2. In a metal bowl, whisk together the egg yolks, sugar, and salt. Pour in the coconut milk, whisking to combine.

3. Pour the mixture back into the saucepan and cook until it is slightly thickened; strain the egg mixture through a mesh sieve into a bowl. Whisk in the vanilla extract.

4. Heat the chocolate in a double boiler over medium-low heat until melted. Stir until the chocolate is smooth and remove it from the heat.

5. Whisk the cooked egg mixture into the chocolate and stir until smooth.

6. Beat the remaining 1¼ cups of the coconut milk until stiff peaks form. Fold the whipped coconut milk into the chocolate mixture.

7. Spoon the mousse into four dessert cups. Chill until ready to serve, at least 3 hours.

Cherry Walnut Bread Pudding

SERVES 8

If you haven't tried bread pudding before, you are in for a treat. This dessert is tender and creamy, filled with delicious cherry and walnut flavor.

FOR THE CUSTARD:
COOKING SPRAY
4 EGGS
4 EGG WHITES
1 CUP SKIM MILK
½ CUP SUGAR
1 TABLESPOON VANILLA EXTRACT
½ TEASPOON GROUND CINNAMON
FOR THE FILLING:
4 CUPS CUBED WHOLE-GRAIN BREAD
2 CUPS PITTED CHERRIES
½ CUP CHOPPED WALNUTS

To make the custard:

1. Preheat the oven to 375°F.

2. Grease a 2-quart casserole dish with cooking spray.

3. Whisk together the eggs, egg whites, and milk in a bowl. Whisk in the sugar, vanilla, and cinnamon until smooth.

To make the filling:

1. Toss together the cubed bread, cherries, and ¼ cup of chopped walnuts in a bowl. Fold in the custard.

2. Transfer the mixture to the casserole dish, pressing down to compact. Cover it with foil.

3. Bake the pudding for 40 to 45 minutes, or until it has set. Remove the foil and sprinkle the pudding with the remaining 1/4 cup of chopped walnuts.

4. Bake for another 15 to 20 minutes, or until the pudding is puffy and golden. Cool the pudding for 15 minutes before serving.

Strawberry Banana Parfaits

SERVES 4

These parfaits are sweet and simple. What more do you need in a dessert?

8 TABLESPOONS WHOLE-GRAIN GRANOLA
2 CUPS VANILLA NONFAT GREEK YOGURT
2 BANANAS, SLICED
16 TABLESPOONS DICED STRAWBERRIES

1. Spoon 1 tablespoon of granola into each of four parfait glasses. Top with ¼ cup of yogurt.

2. Add several slices of banana and 2 tablespoons of diced strawberries to each glass.

3. Top each glass with ¼ cup of yogurt and 1 tablespoon of granola.

4. Finish the parfaits off with the remaining sliced bananas and diced strawberries.

CHAPTER SIX

Week Four

The Mediterranean diet is often considered one of the world's healthiest . . . Dishes mainly feature whole grains, healthier fats . . . and lots of fruit and fresh veggies . . . Several scientific studies have associated this diet with extended life expectancy and lowering risks for heart disease and cancer.

—Toby Amidor, Food Network

WEEK FOUR MEAL PLAN

Day One

Breakfast: Cinnamon Banana Pancakes
Lunch: Basmati Rice Salad with Cranberries
Dinner: Balsamic Salmon with Cherry Tomatoes
Snacks: 2 tablespoons toasted chickpeas; 1 dark chocolate square
Dessert: Tropical Fruit Parfaits

> **Daily Tip:** Try serving today's meals on smaller plates. Using a smaller plate will make the portions appear larger, and you may end up eating less as a result.

Day Two

Breakfast: Maple Walnut Oatmeal
Lunch: Asparagus Leek Risotto
Dinner: Pasta Puttanesca
Snacks: 30 shelled pistachios; 1 cup chopped watermelon
Dessert: Creamy Avocado Sorbet

Daily Tip: Keep your snacks out of sight until you are hungry and need to eat something. If your snacks are readily available, you may eat them simply because you are bored.

Day Three

Breakfast: Cranberry Banana Smoothie
Lunch: Heirloom Tomato Salad
Dinner: Greek-Style Roasted Chicken with Peppers
Snacks: 3 peeled clementines; 4 whole-grain crackers
Dessert: Candied Walnuts

Daily Tip: Try to get in your daily exercise by engaging in activities you like. Take a dance class or a walk through the park, or go on a bike ride with your kids.

Day Four

Breakfast: Mixed Vegetable Frittata
Lunch: Plum Tomato Gazpacho
Dinner: Whole-Grain Pasta with Garlic Artichokes
Snacks: ½ cup fruit salad; 1 sliced apple with 2 teaspoons peanut butter
Dessert: Honey-Poached Pears

Daily Tip: Consider trying out herbal remedies for things like headaches, brittle nails, and more. Check your local health food store for essential oils you can try.

Day Five

Breakfast: Cinnamon Zucchini Bread
Lunch: Rosemary Chicken Panini
Dinner: Grilled Shrimp Skewers
Snacks: 1 sliced kiwi; 3 cups air-popped popcorn
Dessert: Maple Date Truffles

Daily Tip: Use a pedometer to track your daily movements. You can make it a fun challenge for the whole family to beat your step count from the day before.

Day Six

Breakfast: Herbed Cherry Tomato Omelet
Lunch: Red Potato Leek Soup
Dinner: Fresh Basil Pesto Pasta
Snacks: ½ ounce turkey jerky; 1 cup chopped pineapple
Dessert: Lemon Cranberry Scones

Daily Tip: Getting enough sleep is very important for weight loss. Make sure you are getting seven to eight hours a night of restful sleep.

Day Seven

Breakfast: Whole-Grain Banana Nut Muffins
Lunch: Halibut and Arugula Sandwich
Dinner: Fish and White Bean Stew
Snacks: 2 tablespoons hummus with 8 baby carrots; ⅛ ounce sliced avocado
Dessert: Homemade Lemon Pudding

Daily Tip: Drink a mug of green tea with breakfast. Green tea contains powerful antioxidants that can improve your health.

Note: The snacks included in this meal plan are simple snacks you can purchase from the grocery store that need little to no preparation. For more information regarding the nutritional content of these snacks, refer to Appendix A.

ADDITIONAL TIPS FOR WEEK FOUR:

- To encourage restful sleep, stop watching TV and turn off the computer at least one hour before bedtime. Dim lighting will help signal to your body that it's time to wind down.
- When cooking, it can be tempting to take little bites here and there to test the recipe. To cut down on this behavior (and avoid excess calories), try chewing gum while you bake.
- Brush your teeth right after dessert. Not only does this encourage good dental hygiene, but it may also keep you from snacking in the evening.

WEEK FOUR SHOPPING LIST

To prepare your meals for this week, purchase the following items in the quantities indicated:

Pantry Items

- Bay leaf
- Cinnamon, ground
- Cinnamon stick
- Cumin, ground
- Oregano, dried
- Nutmeg, ground
- Pepper
- Rosemary, dried
- Salt
- Canola oil
- Coconut oil

- Cooking spray
- Olive oil, extra-virgin
- Vanilla extract
- Baking powder
- Baking soda
- Cornstarch
- Vinegar, red wine
- Honey
- Maple syrup
- Dijon mustard
- Garlic

Produce

- Basil (2 bunches)
- Cilantro (1 bunch)
- Dill (1 bunch)
- Parsley (1 bunch)
- Rosemary (3 sprigs)
- Thyme (1 bunch)
- Bananas (5)
- Kiwi (1)
- Lemons (3)
- Lime (1)
- Mango (1)
- Pears (4)
- Pineapple chunks (1 cup)
- Arugula (2 cups)
- Asparagus (1 bunch)
- Avocados (2)

- Bell pepper, orange (1)
- Bell pepper, yellow (1)
- Bell peppers, red (4)
- Cucumber, seedless (1 small)
- Leeks (7 small)
- Onion, red (1)
- Onions (4 medium)
- Potatoes, red (3 medium)
- Shallots (4)
- Spinach, baby (6 ounces)
- Tomatoes (2 pounds)
- Tomatoes, cherry (7 pints)
- Tomatoes, heirloom (4 pounds)
- Tomatoes, plum (2 pounds)
- Zucchini (3 medium)
- White mushrooms (1 cup)

Protein

- Bacon (2 slices)
- Chicken, whole, roasting (one, 3½ to 4 pounds)
- Chicken cutlets, boneless (four, 4 to 5 ounces each)
- Halibut fillets (two, 6 ounces; plus 1½ pounds)
- Salmon fillets (four, 4 to 6 ounces each)
- Shrimp, raw (1 pound)

Dairy

- Almond milk, unsweetened (2 cups)
- Coconut milk, unsweetened (1 cup)
- Half-and-half (1 cup)
- Milk, skim (6 cups)
- Mozzarella cheese (1 pound)
- Mozzarella cheese, shredded (1 cup)
- Parmesan cheese, grated (½ cup)
- Mayonnaise, olive oil (¼ cup)
- Yogurt, plain nonfat Greek (1½ cups)
- Yogurt, vanilla nonfat Greek (2 cups)

Dry Foods

- Flour, unbleached (2 cups)
- Flour, whole-wheat (4 cups)
- Sugar (3¼ cups)
- Oats, rolled (1 cup)
- Oats, steel-cut (1 cup)
- Rice, arborio (1 cup)
- Rice, basmati (2 cups)
- Linguine, whole-wheat (8 ounces)
- Penne, whole-wheat (12 ounces)
- Rotini, whole-wheat (12 ounces)
- Beans, white cannellini (two 15-ounce cans)
- Cranberries, dried (1½ cups)
- Dates, pitted (1⅓ cups)
- Raisins (1 cup)
- Granola, whole-grain (½ cup)
- Almonds, sliced (1 cup)
- Cashews (1 cup)
- Pine nuts (1 tablespoon)
- Walnut halves (1½ cups)
- Walnuts, chopped (¼ cup)

Refrigerated and Frozen Foods

- Eggs (22)
- Cranberry juice (¼ cup)

- Bananas, frozen (2)
- Cranberries, frozen (1 cup)

Other

- Bread, ciabatta (1 loaf)
- Bread, Italian (1 loaf)
- Applesauce, unsweetened (1 cup)
- Artichoke hearts, marinated (1 can)
- Black olives, halved (¼ cup)
- Black olives, sliced (½ cup)
- Capers (¼ cup)
- Kalamata olives, sliced (¼ cup)
- Roasted garlic dressing (1 cup)

- Sun-dried tomatoes in oil (½ cup)
- Tomatoes, diced (one 14.5-ounce can)
- Tomatoes, slow-roasted (1 cup)
- Clam juice (1 cup)
- Sherry, dry (¼ cup)
- White wine, dry (1 cup)
- Broth, vegetable (4 cups)
- Wooden skewers

PLAN-AHEAD PREPARATIONS

This week there are several things you can prepare ahead of time and use throughout the week to make your life easier.

1. **Sliced black olives:** You will use these in several recipes. If you prefer not to buy pre-sliced olives, purchase them whole and slice them yourself using a small, sharp knife.
2. **Sliced vegetables:** You can never have enough sliced vegetables on hand. This week you will use sliced vegetables in various salads as well as in a Plum Tomato Gazpacho and Mixed Vegetable Frittata. You can use whatever vegetables you like, but some recommendations include zucchini, broccoli, carrots, mushrooms, tomatoes, and summer squash.
3. **Fresh lemon juice:** Lemon juice will be used in several recipes this week. Juice several lemons at a time and store the juice in an airtight container in the fridge.

4. **Overripe bananas:** On Day Seven you will enjoy Whole-Grain Banana Nut Muffins for breakfast. In order to prepare this recipe, you will need a few bananas that are very ripe. For best results, purchase the bananas early in the week and let them sit out on the counter until the peels begin to darken with spots.

5. **Avocados:** For dessert on Day Two you will enjoy Creamy Avocado Sorbet. For best results, the avocados you use should be ripe. Purchase your avocados early in the week and if they are not yet ripe, store them in a paper bag on the kitchen counter to soften them up a bit.

WEEK FOUR RECIPES

Breakfast Recipes

CINNAMON BANANA PANCAKES

MAPLE WALNUT OATMEAL

CRANBERRY BANANA SMOOTHIE

MIXED VEGETABLE FRITTATA

CINNAMON ZUCCHINI BREAD

HERBED CHERRY TOMATO OMELET

WHOLE-GRAIN BANANA NUT MUFFINS

Lunch Recipes

BASMATI RICE SALAD WITH CRANBERRIES

ASPARAGUS LEEK RISOTTO

HEIRLOOM TOMATO SALAD

PLUM TOMATO GAZPACHO

ROSEMARY CHICKEN PANINI

RED POTATO LEEK SOUP

HALIBUT AND ARUGULA SANDWICH

Dinner Recipes

BALSAMIC SALMON WITH CHERRY TOMATOES

PASTA PUTTANESCA

GREEK-STYLE ROASTED CHICKEN WITH PEPPERS

WHOLE-GRAIN PASTA WITH GARLIC ARTICHOKES

GRILLED SHRIMP SKEWERS

FRESH BASIL PESTO PASTA

FISH AND WHITE BEAN STEW

Dessert Recipes

TROPICAL FRUIT PARFAITS

CREAMY AVOCADO SORBET

CANDIED WALNUTS

HONEY-POACHED PEARS

MAPLE DATE TRUFFLES

LEMON CRANBERRY SCONES

HOMEMADE LEMON PUDDING

Cinnamon Banana Pancakes

SERVES 4

These pancakes are sure to be a hit with the whole family. Drizzle them with maple syrup or top them with a few slices of fresh banana.

1 CUP SKIM MILK
1 CUP WHOLE-WHEAT FLOUR
1 EGG
1 BANANA, SLICED
1 TABLESPOON HONEY
1 TABLESPOON COCONUT OIL, MELTED
1 TEASPOON VANILLA EXTRACT
1 TEASPOON GROUND CINNAMON
1½ TEASPOONS BAKING POWDER
COOKING SPRAY

1. Combine all the ingredients in a blender and blend on high speed for 30 seconds, or until smooth. Let sit for 5 minutes.

2. Grease a heavy skillet with cooking spray and heat it over medium-high heat.

3. Spoon the batter about ¼ cup at a time onto the hot skillet. Cook the pancakes until bubbles appear on the surface, about 2 to 3 minutes.

4. Flip the pancakes and cook for 1 to 2 minutes, or until lightly browned underneath. Slide the pancakes onto a plate and repeat with the remaining batter.

5. Serve hot, drizzled with syrup.

Maple Walnut Oatmeal

SERVES 4

This nutty oatmeal is a hot and hearty way to start your day. Studies show that if you start your day with a good breakfast, you will be less likely to snack between meals.

2 CUPS WATER

1 CUP STEEL-CUT OATS

⅓ CUP RAISINS

¼ TEASPOON GROUND CINNAMON

PINCH OF SALT

1 TABLESPOON MAPLE SYRUP

¼ CUP CHOPPED WALNUTS

1. Whisk together the water and steel-cut oats in a small saucepan over medium heat.

2. Add the raisins, cinnamon, and salt.

3. Bring to a boil, then reduce the heat and simmer on low, uncovered, for about 20 minutes.

4. Spoon the oatmeal into bowls and top with chopped walnuts and a drizzle of maple syrup to serve.

Cranberry Banana Smoothie

SERVES 2

A smoothie is a quick and easy breakfast for people on the go—simply pour it into a travel mug and you are out the door.

2 FROZEN BANANAS, SLICED
1 CUP FROZEN CRANBERRIES
1 CUP SKIM MILK
½ CUP PLAIN NONFAT GREEK YOGURT
¼ CUP CRANBERRY JUICE
2 TABLESPOONS HONEY

1. Combine all the ingredients in a blender. Blend for 30 seconds on high, or until smooth.

2. Pour the smoothie into two glasses and serve immediately.

Mixed Vegetable Frittata

SERVES 6

This mixed vegetable frittata is the perfect family breakfast on the weekend. One recipe serves everyone and gets you on your way to the rest of your weekend plans.

1 CUP CHOPPED WHITE MUSHROOMS
½ CUP CHOPPED ZUCCHINI
¼ CUP CHOPPED ONION
¼ CUP CHOPPED RED BELL PEPPER
1 TABLESPOON EXTRA-VIRGIN OLIVE OIL
½ TEASPOON DRIED OREGANO
SALT AND FRESHLY GROUND PEPPER
⅓ CUP SHREDDED MOZZARELLA CHEESE
8 EGGS, BEATEN
2 TABLESPOONS GRATED PARMESAN CHEESE

1. Preheat the broiler to high heat.

2. Heat the olive oil in an ovenproof skillet over medium heat. Add the mushrooms and vegetables and toss to coat with oil.

3. Cook the mushrooms and vegetables for 2 minutes; stir in the oregano, and season with salt and pepper. Cook for 6 to 7 minutes more, or until the mushrooms and vegetables are tender.

4. Reduce the heat to low and sprinkle the mozzarella over the zucchini. Pour in the beaten eggs and stir gently.

5. Cover the skillet and cook on low for 15 minutes, or until the frittata is almost set.

6. Uncover the skillet and place it under the broiler for 2 minutes, until browned. Sprinkle the frittata with the grated Parmesan and let it sit for 5 minutes before serving.

Cinnamon Zucchini Bread

MAKES 1 LOAF

Flavored with cinnamon and a hint of zucchini, this bread is more than just a breakfast—it is a treat.

COOKING SPRAY

½ CUP CANOLA OIL

2 EGGS

1 CUP SUGAR

¼ CUP SKIM MILK

1 TEASPOON VANILLA EXTRACT

1 CUP WHOLE-WHEAT FLOUR

1 CUP UNBLEACHED FLOUR

1 TEASPOON BAKING SODA

½ TEASPOON BAKING POWDER

½ TEASPOON SALT

2 TEASPOONS GROUND CINNAMON

2 CUPS GRATED ZUCCHINI

1. Preheat the oven to 350°F.

2. Lightly grease a regular loaf pan with cooking spray.

3. Whisk together the canola oil, eggs, sugar, milk, and vanilla extract in a large mixing bowl.

4. In a separate bowl, stir together the flours, baking soda, baking powder, salt, and cinnamon.

5. Stir the dry ingredients into the wet ingredients until the mixture is well combined. Fold in the zucchini.

6. Spoon the batter into the prepared pan and bake for 60 to 75 minutes, or until a knife inserted in the center of the loaf comes out clean.

7. Remove the loaf from the oven and let it stand for 10 minutes. Turn the loaf out onto a wire rack to cool completely before cutting.

Herbed Cherry Tomato Omelet

SERVES 2

Slicing the cherry tomatoes in half allows their juice to soak into the egg in this flavorful omelet.

2 EGGS

1 TABLESPOON SKIM MILK

½ TEASPOON SALT

¼ TEASPOON FRESHLY GROUND PEPPER

2 TEASPOONS EXTRA-VIRGIN OLIVE OIL

½ CUP HALVED CHERRY TOMATOES

2 TABLESPOONS CHOPPED FRESH BASIL

2 TABLESPOONS CHOPPED FRESH PARSLEY

1 SMALL SHALLOT, DICED

1. Crack the eggs into a small bowl and whisk in the skim milk, salt, and pepper until well combined. Set the bowl aside.

2. Heat 1 teaspoon of olive oil in a small skillet over medium heat.

3. Stir in the tomatoes, herbs, and shallot and cook for 2 to 3 minutes, or until hot.

4. Spoon the tomato mixture into a bowl and set aside.

5. Heat the remaining teaspoon of olive oil in the same skillet and pour in the egg mixture. Rotate the pan to coat the sides with egg.

6. Let the eggs cook for 1 minute; then scrape down the sides of the pan using a spatula, letting the uncooked egg spread.

7. Allow the eggs to cook for 1 to 2 minutes longer, or until almost set. Spoon the tomato mixture over half the omelet.

8. Fold the empty half of the omelet over the tomato filling and allow the eggs to cook for 1 more minute, or until the eggs are cooked through. Serve hot.

Whole-Grain Banana Nut Muffins

MAKES 12 MUFFINS

Banana and walnut are two flavors that are just meant to be together—the evidence is in this recipe.

1 CUP ROLLED OATS

1 CUP WHOLE-WHEAT FLOUR

1 TEASPOON GROUND CINNAMON

1 TEASPOON BAKING SODA

½ TEASPOON SALT

3 BANANAS, MASHED

½ CUP HONEY

2 EGGS

1 TEASPOON VANILLA EXTRACT

1. Preheat the oven to 325°F.

2. Combine the oats, flour, cinnamon, baking soda, and salt in a medium mixing bowl and stir well.

3. In a separate mixing bowl, beat the bananas, honey, eggs, and vanilla extract until smooth.

4. Add the dry ingredients to the wet ingredients in small batches, stirring until smooth after each addition.

5. Line a muffin tin with paper liners and fill each cup about two-thirds full with batter.

6. Bake the muffins for 20 to 25 minutes, or until a knife inserted in the center comes out clean.

7. Cool the muffins in the pan for 5 minutes, then turn them out onto a wire cooling rack to cool completely before serving.

Basmati Rice Salad with Cranberries

SERVES 6

If you are tired of eating sandwiches for lunch, give this basmati rice salad a try. Flavored with fresh cilantro and parsley, and studded with cranberries, this recipe will have you loving lunch again.

1 TEASPOON EXTRA-VIRGIN OLIVE OIL

1 CUP SLICED ALMONDS

2 CUPS BASMATI RICE

3 CUPS WATER

1 CUP UNSWEETENED COCONUT MILK

½ CUP DRIED CRANBERRIES

½ CUP RAISINS

¼ CUP CHOPPED FRESH CILANTRO

2 TABLESPOONS CHOPPED FRESH PARSLEY

1 TABLESPOON LEMON ZEST

SALT AND FRESHLY GROUND PEPPER

1. Heat the oil in a skillet over medium heat. Add the almonds and toss to coat.

2. Toast the almonds until they are lightly browned, about 2 to 3 minutes, stirring often. Drain the almonds on a paper towel.

3. Combine the basmati rice, water, and coconut milk in a saucepan. Stir well, and cover the rice mixture with the lid.

4. Cook the rice until the water has been absorbed and the rice is tender, about 20 minutes.

5. Spoon the rice into a serving bowl and stir in the remaining ingredients. Serve warm.

Asparagus Leek Risotto

SERVES 4

This risotto is the ultimate in indulgent lunches. Hot and creamy, with just enough leek and asparagus flavor, it will soon be a favorite.

1 BUNCH ASPARAGUS SPEARS, TRIMMED

4 CUPS HOT WATER

1 TABLESPOON EXTRA-VIRGIN OLIVE OIL

½ CUP DICED LEEK

1 CUP ARBORIO RICE

½ CUP DRY WHITE WINE

CHOPPED FRESH PARSLEY, FOR GARNISH

To Blanch the Asparagus:

1. Cut the asparagus diagonally about 3 inches below the tip.

2. Place the asparagus in a skillet and heat over medium heat. Add 2 tablespoons of water and bring to a boil to blanch the asparagus.

3. Cook the asparagus only until it is bright green (about 2 to 4 minutes), then plunge it into an ice-water bath to stop the cooking. Set aside.

4. Bring the 4 cups of hot water to a boil in a saucepan. Set aside, keeping the water hot over medium-low heat.

5. Heat the oil in a medium saucepan and stir in the leek. Cook for 2 minutes, then stir in the arborio rice and stir to coat with oil.

6. Cook the rice for 3 to 5 minutes, then stir in the wine. Cook until most of the liquid has cooked off.

7. Stir in 1 cup of hot water and bring to a simmer. Reduce the heat and simmer for 8 minutes, stirring often.

continued ▶

8. Once most of the liquid has been absorbed, add the remaining 3 cups of water 1 cup at a time, simmering and stirring until each addition has been absorbed, about 15 minutes total.

9. After the final addition, stir in the asparagus. Cover and remove the rice from the heat. Set aside for 5 minutes.

10. Spoon the risotto into serving bowls and garnish with parsley to serve.

Heirloom Tomato Salad

SERVES 6 TO 8

If you like your lunches a little on the lighter side, this heirloom tomato salad is just what you've been looking for.

½ CUP EXTRA-VIRGIN OLIVE OIL

2 TABLESPOONS RED WINE VINEGAR

1 TEASPOON DIJON MUSTARD

1 TEASPOON SALT

½ TEASPOON FRESH GROUND PEPPER

½ TEASPOON SUGAR

4 POUNDS HEIRLOOM TOMATOES, CUT INTO WEDGES

1 PINT CHERRY TOMATOES

1 POUND FRESH MOZZARELLA, CUT INTO ¼-INCH CHUNKS

1½ CUPS PACKED FRESH BASIL LEAVES, TORN INTO CHUNKS

1. Whisk together the olive oil, vinegar, mustard, salt, pepper, and sugar until well combined.

2. Combine the remaining ingredients in a mixing bowl and toss with the dressing to coat.

3. Chill until ready to serve.

Plum Tomato Gazpacho

SERVES 6

Tomato gazpacho is a classic recipe typically enjoyed during the summer using fresh produce. You can make it all year round, however, so don't limit yourself to just one season of enjoyment.

2 POUNDS PLUM TOMATOES, HALVED
1 RED BELL PEPPER, SEEDED AND COARSELY CHOPPED
1 CUP CHOPPED RED ONION
1 CUP CHOPPED SEEDLESS CUCUMBER
¼ CUP DRY SHERRY
¼ CUP EXTRA-VIRGIN OLIVE OIL
1 TEASPOON MINCED GARLIC
½ TEASPOON GROUND CUMIN
1 CUP WATER
SALT AND FRESHLY GROUND PEPPER

1. Over a mixing bowl, use your hands to squeeze the seeds and juices out of the halved tomatoes. Extract as much moisture as possible.

2. Strain the juice and discard the seeds. Chop the tomatoes and stir them into the juice in the mixing bowl.

3. Stir in the remaining ingredients except for the water, salt, and pepper, and let it sit for 1 hour.

4. Blend the gazpacho in batches in a blender until smooth, using the water as needed to thin.

5. Season the soup with salt and pepper and chill for at least 2 hours before serving.

Rosemary Chicken Panini

SERVES 4

This chicken panini will have your mouth watering before you even take the first bite. From start to finish, this recipe is one you are going to enjoy.

FOUR 4- TO 5-OUNCE BONELESS CHICKEN CUTLETS

2 TABLESPOONS EXTRA-VIRGIN OLIVE OIL

1 TEASPOON CHOPPED FRESH ROSEMARY

1 TABLESPOON MINCED GARLIC

¼ CUP CHOPPED SUN-DRIED TOMATOES IN OIL

6 OUNCES FRESH BABY SPINACH

SALT AND FRESHLY GROUND PEPPER

COOKING SPRAY

8 TABLESPOONS (ABOUT 2 OUNCES) SHREDDED MOZZARELLA CHEESE

1 LOAF ITALIAN BREAD, CUT INTO 8 SLICES

1. Place the chicken cutlets in a zippered freezer bag. Add 1 tablespoon of olive oil and the chopped rosemary and toss to coat.

2. Seal the bag and chill for 30 minutes.

3. Heat the remaining tablespoon of oil in a skillet over medium-high heat. Add the garlic and cook for 1 minute.

4. Stir in the sun-dried tomatoes and cook for 1 minute more.

5. Add the spinach and cook until wilted, about 1 minute.

6. Season the sun-dried tomatoes and spinach with salt and pepper.

7. Heat a stovetop grill pan over medium-high heat and coat it with cooking spray. Place the chicken cutlets on the grill and cook for 3 minutes on each side, or until cooked through.

continued ▶

8. Spoon about 1 tablespoon of mozzarella cheese onto each of 4 slices of bread and top with 1 chicken cutlet each.

9. Place one-fourth of the spinach mixture on top of each chicken cutlet and top with another tablespoon of cheese. Top with another slice of bread.

10. Reheat the grill pan and coat it with cooking spray.

11. Place 2 sandwiches on the pan and press flat with a heavy lid or skillet. Cook for 3 to 4 minutes on each side, or until toasted.

12. Repeat the process with the remaining 2 sandwiches and serve warm.

Red Potato Leek Soup

Hot and creamy, this potato soup is the perfect lunch to enjoy in cool weather. Even if it isn't cold out, you can pretend it is by putting on a sweater and spooning up a bowl of this delicious soup.

2 TABLESPOONS EXTRA-VIRGIN OLIVE OIL

1 TABLESPOON MINCED GARLIC

1 CUP CHOPPED ONIONS

3 LEEKS, CHOPPED (WHITE AND LIGHT GREEN PARTS ONLY)

SALT AND FRESHLY GROUND PEPPER

3 MEDIUM RED POTATOES, CHOPPED

1 BAY LEAF

4 CUPS VEGETABLE BROTH

2 CUPS UNSWEETENED ALMOND MILK

1 TABLESPOON CHOPPED FRESH DILL

1. Heat the oil in a stockpot over medium heat. Add the garlic and cook for 1 minute.

2. Stir in the onions and leeks, season them with salt and pepper, and cook for 6 to 8 minutes, or until the onions are tender.

3. Stir in the potatoes, bay leaf, and vegetable broth. Bring to a boil, then reduce the heat and simmer for 35 minutes.

4. Stir in the almond milk and dill and simmer for 5 minutes longer.

5. Discard the bay leaf and serve hot.

Halibut and Arugula Sandwich

SERVES 4

Step outside the norm of ham and cheese sandwiches with this halibut sandwich. It is easy to prepare the halibut the night before so you can whip this sandwich up fresh before heading to work in the morning.

COOKING SPRAY

TWO 6-OUNCE HALIBUT FILLETS, SKIN REMOVED

SALT AND FRESHLY GROUND PEPPER

2 TABLESPOONS PLUS 1 TEASPOON EXTRA-VIRGIN OLIVE OIL

1 LOAF CIABATTA BREAD, CUT INTO 8 SLICES

¼ CUP OLIVE OIL MAYONNAISE

¼ CUP CHOPPED SUN-DRIED TOMATOES IN OIL

3 TABLESPOONS CHOPPED FRESH BASIL

2 TABLESPOONS CHOPPED FRESH PARSLEY

1 TABLESPOON CAPERS, RINSED AND DRAINED

2 CUPS ARUGULA

1. Preheat the oven to 450°F.

2. Lightly grease a baking sheet with cooking spray and add the halibut. Season the halibut with salt and pepper and rub with 1 teaspoon of the oil.

3. Bake the halibut for 10 to 12 minutes, or until the fish flakes easily with a fork. Set aside to cool.

4. Brush the slices of bread with oil and place them on a baking sheet. Bake the bread for 6 to 8 minutes, or until it is just browned.

5. Combine the remaining ingredients except the arugula in a bowl and stir well. Add the fish, flaking it into the bowl with a fork.

6. Stir well, then spoon the mixture onto 4 slices of toasted bread. Top each slice with a handful of arugula and another piece of bread to serve.

Balsamic Salmon with Cherry Tomatoes

SERVES 4

After a long day at work, the last thing you want is to come home and spend an hour preparing dinner. This balsamic salmon recipe is quick and easy, but definitely not lacking in flavor.

COOKING SPRAY

2 PINTS CHERRY TOMATOES, HALVED

1 TABLESPOON EXTRA-VIRGIN OLIVE OIL

1 TABLESPOON MINCED GARLIC

2 TEASPOONS FRESH CHOPPED THYME

½ TEASPOON SALT

½ TEASPOON FRESHLY GROUND PEPPER

FOUR 4- TO 6-OUNCE SALMON FILLETS

1. Preheat the oven to 400°F.

2. Spray a rimmed baking sheet with cooking spray.

3. Combine the cherry tomatoes with the olive oil, garlic, thyme, salt, and pepper in a mixing bowl. Spread the mixture on the baking sheet.

4. Roast the tomato mixture for 15 minutes, then remove it from the oven.

5. Arrange the salmon fillets in a square glass baking dish and top with the tomato mixture.

6. Bake the salmon for 10 minutes, or until the fish flakes easily with a fork. Serve hot.

Pasta Puttanesca

SERVES 6

This pasta dish utilizes all your favorite Mediterranean flavors, from garlic and tomato to capers and olives, in one fantastic dish.

2 POUNDS TOMATOES, QUARTERED

1 TABLESPOON MINCED GARLIC

3 TABLESPOONS CAPERS, RINSED WELL

2 TABLESPOONS EXTRA-VIRGIN OLIVE OIL

SALT AND FRESHLY GROUND PEPPER

¼ CUP SLICED KALAMATA OLIVES

12 OUNCES WHOLE-GRAIN PENNE

1. Preheat the oven to 425°F.

2. Combine the tomatoes, garlic, and capers in a mixing bowl. Toss with the olive oil, season with salt and pepper, and spread the mixture on a baking sheet.

3. Roast the tomato mixture for 35 minutes, then reduce the oven temperature to 375°F. Stir in the olives and roast for 15 minutes more.

4. Bring a pot of salted water to boil and cook the pasta al dente according to the package directions. Drain the pasta and set aside.

5. Stir the roasted tomato mixture into the cooked pasta. Season with salt and pepper to serve.

Greek-Style Roasted Chicken with Peppers

SERVES 4 TO 6

If you are looking for the perfect recipe to share with friends and family, try this Greek-style roasted chicken. Full of flavor and accompanied by tender peppers, this chicken is sure to be a hit.

ONE 3½- TO 4-POUND ROASTING CHICKEN

1 LEMON, HALVED

2 SPRIGS FRESH ROSEMARY

SALT

3 LEEKS, WASHED, TRIMMED, AND CHOPPED

2 RED BELL PEPPERS, SEEDED AND CHOPPED

1 YELLOW BELL PEPPER, SEEDED AND CHOPPED

1 ORANGE BELL PEPPER, SEEDED AND CHOPPED

½ CUP SLICED BLACK OLIVES

¼ CUP EXTRA-VIRGIN OLIVE OIL

1 TABLESPOON DRIED ROSEMARY

FRESHLY GROUND PEPPER

1. Preheat the oven to 400°F.

2. Remove the giblet bag from the cavity of the chicken and rinse the chicken well with cool water. Pat the chicken dry inside and out with paper towels.

3. Place the chicken in a roasting pan and stuff the lemon and fresh rosemary into the cavity. Season the chicken with salt.

4. Combine the leeks, bell peppers, and olives in a mixing bowl and toss with the olive oil. Season with dried rosemary, salt, and pepper.

5. Pour the vegetables into the roasting pan around the chicken.

continued ▶

6. Roast the chicken and vegetables for 1 hour and 15 minutes, or until the chicken's juices run clear.

7. Remove the chicken to a cutting board and let it rest for 10 minutes. Return the roasting pan with the vegetables to the oven and turn off the heat.

8. Carve the chicken as desired and serve with the vegetables.

Whole-Grain Pasta with Garlic Artichokes

SERVES 4

Artichokes are naturally high in antioxidants and have been shown to reduce the risk of cancer. If you are looking for a recipe that is as healthful as it is delicious, look no further.

SALT

12 OUNCES WHOLE-WHEAT ROTINI

2 TABLESPOONS EXTRA-VIRGIN OLIVE OIL

1 TEASPOON MINCED GARLIC

1 CUP CHOPPED ONION

½ CUP DRY WHITE WINE

ONE 14-OUNCE CAN ARTICHOKE HEARTS, DRAINED, RINSED,
   AND QUARTERED

¼ CUP HALVED BLACK OLIVES

2 CUPS HALVED CHERRY TOMATOES

¼ CUP GRATED PARMESAN CHEESE

½ CUP FRESH SLICED BASIL LEAVES

FRESHLY GROUND PEPPER

1. Bring a large pot of salted water to boil. Add the rotini and cook al dente according to the package directions.

2. Drain the pasta, reserving 1 cup of liquid.

3. Heat 1 tablespoon of olive oil in a skillet over medium-high heat. Add the garlic and cook for 1 minute.

4. Stir in the onion and cook for 3 to 4 minutes.

5. Add the wine and cook until it has evaporated, 2 to 3 minutes.

6. Add the artichokes and cook for 2 to 3 minutes, or until they are lightly browned.

continued ▶

7. Stir in the olives and tomatoes. Cook for 1 to 2 minutes.

8. Stir the cooked pasta into the skillet and add the remaining tablespoon of olive oil along with the Parmesan cheese and basil.

9. If needed, thin the sauce with the reserved cooking water. Season with salt and pepper, and serve.

Grilled Shrimp Skewers

SERVES 4

These grilled shrimp are perfect for a summer meal. Enjoy them on the patio with friends, accompanied by a nice glass of wine.

WOODEN SKEWERS
1 POUND LARGE RAW SHRIMP, PEELED AND DEVEINED
SALT AND FRESHLY GROUND PEPPER
1 CUP STORE-BOUGHT ROASTED GARLIC DRESSING
1 TABLESPOON FRESH LEMON JUICE
COOKING SPRAY

1. Soak the skewers in water for 30 minutes to prevent them from burning on the grill.

2. Slide the shrimp onto the skewers through both ends of each shrimp. Place the skewers in a shallow dish and season with salt and pepper.

3. Whisk together the garlic dressing and lemon juice in a bowl; pour the dressing over the shrimp. Turn the shrimp to make sure they are all coated.

4. Chill the shrimp for 20 to 25 minutes.

5. Preheat the grill to medium-high heat.

6. Lightly grease the grill grates with cooking spray.

7. Place the shrimp skewers on the grill and cover. Cook for 2 to 3 minutes, then turn the skewers.

8. Cover the grill again and cook for 2 to 3 minutes more, or until the shrimp is cooked through. Serve hot.

Fresh Basil Pesto Pasta

SERVES 4

What makes this pasta special is the homemade basil pesto. You may find yourself loving this recipe so much that you plant an entire garden of basil next spring.

FOR THE PESTO:

1 GARLIC CLOVE, PEELED

1 TABLESPOON PINE NUTS

PINCH OF SALT

1½ CUPS PACKED FRESH BASIL

¼ CUP EXTRA-VIRGIN OLIVE OIL

2 TABLESPOONS GRATED PARMESAN CHEESE

FOR THE PASTA:

SALT

8 OUNCES WHOLE-WHEAT LINGUINE

1 CUP CANNED SLOW-ROASTED TOMATOES, WITH JUICES

FRESHLY GROUND PEPPER

GRATED PARMESAN CHEESE, FOR GARNISH

To make the pesto:

1. Combine the garlic, pine nuts, and salt in a food processor and blend on high speed for 15 seconds. Add the basil, and pulse to shred.

2. With the processor running, drizzle in the olive oil until smooth. Blend in the Parmesan cheese to finish. Set aside.

To make the pasta:

1. Bring a large pot of salted water to boil. Add the linguine and cook al dente according to the package directions.

2. Drain the pasta, reserving ¼ cup of liquid, and return the pasta to the pot.

3. Add the fresh pesto and stir well over medium-low heat. Add the reserved water a little at a time to create a sauce.

4. Stir in the slow-roasted tomatoes and season with salt and pepper.

5. Heat until cooked through and serve hot, garnished with grated Parmesan cheese.

Fish and White Bean Stew

SERVES 4

This fish stew is simple yet satisfying—hot enough to warm you on the coldest day, and hearty enough to put your hunger to rest.

2 BACON SLICES, CHOPPED

1 CUP DICED SHALLOTS

2 TABLESPOONS EXTRA-VIRGIN OLIVE OIL

1 TABLESPOON MINCED GARLIC

ONE 14.5-OUNCE CAN DICED TOMATOES

1 CUP CLAM JUICE

¼ CUP DRY WHITE WINE

TWO 15-OUNCE CANS WHITE CANNELLINI BEANS, DRAINED AND RINSED

1½ POUNDS HALIBUT FILLETS, CUT INTO 2-INCH CHUNKS

SALT AND FRESHLY GROUND PEPPER

1. Heat the chopped bacon and shallots in a large saucepan over medium-high heat. Cook until the bacon is crisp, 6 to 7 minutes.

2. Stir in the olive oil and garlic and cook for 1 minute.

3. Add the diced tomatoes, clam juice, and wine. Bring the mixture to a boil, then reduce the heat and simmer for 5 minutes.

4. Stir in the cannellini beans and fish and bring to a simmer over medium-low heat.

5. Cover and cook until the fish is just cooked through, about 5 minutes. Season with salt and pepper, and serve.

Tropical Fruit Parfaits

SERVES 4

These fruit parfaits are a light and easy way to enjoy dessert. Nothing heavy here—just fruit and yogurt with a sprinkling of granola.

1 BANANA, SLICED

1 MANGO, PITTED AND CHOPPED

1 CUP PINEAPPLE CHUNKS

1 KIWI, PEELED AND CHOPPED

2 CUPS VANILLA NONFAT GREEK YOGURT

½ CUP WHOLE-GRAIN GRANOLA

1. Combine the fruit in a bowl and stir to combine.

2. Spoon 1 tablespoon of fruit into each of four parfait glasses. Top with ¼ cup of yogurt and 1 tablespoon of granola.

3. Add several tablespoons of fruit to each glass.

4. Top each glass with ¼ cup of yogurt and another tablespoon of granola.

5. Finish the parfaits off with the remaining fruit and chill until ready to serve.

Creamy Avocado Sorbet

SERVES 4

This creamy sorbet is like no frozen dessert you have tried before. To make it work, use the freshest avocados you can find.

1 CUP WATER

¼ CUP SUGAR

2 AVOCADOS, PEELED, PITTED, AND CHOPPED

2 TABLESPOONS FRESH LIME JUICE

1 TABLESPOON HONEY

1 TEASPOON LIME ZEST

1. Whisk together the water and sugar in a saucepan over medium heat. Stir until the sugar dissolves.

2. Remove the saucepan from the heat and let it cool.

3. Place the avocados in a food processor and blend until smooth. Add the remaining ingredients and purée.

4. Add the sugar water and blend until smooth.

5. Pour the mixture into a shallow dish; cover and freeze.

6. Just before serving, break the sorbet into chunks and blend in a food processor until smooth.

Candied Walnuts

MAKES 1½ CUPS

If you are looking for a sweet snack or just a little something after dinner, these tasty walnuts are the thing. Lightly toasted and coated in sugar, they are sure to satisfy your sweet tooth.

1½ CUPS WALNUT HALVES
½ CUP SUGAR
PINCH OF SALT

1. Preheat the oven to 350°F.

2. Spread the walnuts on a baking sheet in a single layer and bake for 5 minutes, or until they are lightly toasted.

3. Place the sugar and salt in a heavy-bottomed saucepan and cook over medium heat, stirring often. As soon as the sugar begins to melt, about 2 minutes, start stirring constantly. When it turns amber in color after 2 to 3 minutes more, stir in the walnuts to coat.

4. Spread the walnuts on the baking sheet and sprinkle them with salt. Let the walnuts cool completely before serving.

Honey-Poached Pears

SERVES 4

If you aren't a fan of elaborate desserts, these poached pears may be perfect for you. Poached in cinnamon- and honey-flavored water, these pears are tender and flavorful.

4 CUPS WATER

½ CUP HONEY, PLUS MORE FOR SERVING

2 TABLESPOONS SUGAR

1 CINNAMON STICK, BROKEN IN HALF

4 PEARS, PEELED, HALVED, AND CORED

1. Whisk together the water, honey, and sugar in a saucepan and bring to a boil. Stir until the sugar dissolves, then add the cinnamon stick.

2. Add the pears to the liquid and reduce to a simmer. Cover and cook the pears for 20 to 30 minutes, or until the pears are tender.

3. Remove the pears from the liquid with a slotted spoon, drizzle them with honey, and serve.

Maple Date Truffles

SERVES 6

These truffles are not your average confection. Rather than being loaded with calories and saturated fat, they are made with wholesome ingredients like pitted dates and cashews.

1⅓ CUPS PITTED DATES
1 CUP WHOLE CASHEWS
1 TABLESPOON MAPLE SYRUP
1 TEASPOON VANILLA EXTRACT
PINCH OF SALT

1. Combine all the ingredients in a food processor and blend until they begin to stick together.

2. Roll the mixture into 1-inch balls by hand and place them on a plate. Chill the truffles until ready to serve.

Lemon Cranberry Scones

SERVES 8

If you love to bake, you are definitely going to want to try this scone recipe. In fact, you may find yourself baking them every week.

1 CUP WHOLE-WHEAT FLOUR

1 CUP UNBLEACHED FLOUR

¼ CUP SUGAR

2 TEASPOONS BAKING POWDER

1 TEASPOON GROUND CINNAMON

½ TEASPOON BAKING SODA

¼ TEASPOON GROUND NUTMEG

PINCH OF SALT

¼ CUP COCONUT OIL

1 CUP UNSWEETENED APPLESAUCE

½ CUP PLAIN NONFAT GREEK YOGURT

1 EGG

2 TABLESPOONS LEMON ZEST

1 TEASPOON VANILLA EXTRACT

1 CUP DRIED CRANBERRIES

1. Preheat the oven to 425°F.

2. Line a baking sheet with parchment paper.

3. Combine the dry ingredients, except for the cranberries, in a mixing bowl and blend well. Whisk in the coconut oil and stir until well combined.

4. Add the applesauce, yogurt, egg, lemon zest, and vanilla extract. Stir until just blended. Fold in the cranberries.

5. Turn the dough out onto a floured surface and knead several times. Pat the dough into a circle about ¾-inch thick.

6. Use a sharp knife to cut the circle into 8 triangles, then place them on the baking sheet. Bake for 15 to 18 minutes, or until the scones are golden brown.

7. Cool the scones for 10 minutes before serving.

Homemade Lemon Pudding

SERVES 8

This lemon pudding is cool and creamy with just the right amount of fresh lemon flavor.

6 EGG YOLKS
1 CUP PLUS 2 TABLESPOONS SUGAR
5 TABLESPOONS CORNSTARCH
1 TABLESPOON LEMON ZEST
PINCH OF SALT
3½ CUPS SKIM MILK
1 CUP HALF-AND-HALF
1 CUP FRESH LEMON JUICE

1. Whisk together the egg yolks with 1 cup of sugar, the cornstarch, lemon zest, and salt in a medium saucepan. Whisk in ½ cup of milk until smooth.

2. Gradually add the remaining 3 cups of milk and the half-and-half, whisking until smooth between each addition.

3. Bring the mixture to a simmer, whisking as it heats.

4. Remove the saucepan from heat and whisk in the lemon juice.

5. Strain the pudding through a sieve and discard the solids. Spoon the pudding into dessert cups and chill for 2 hours before serving.

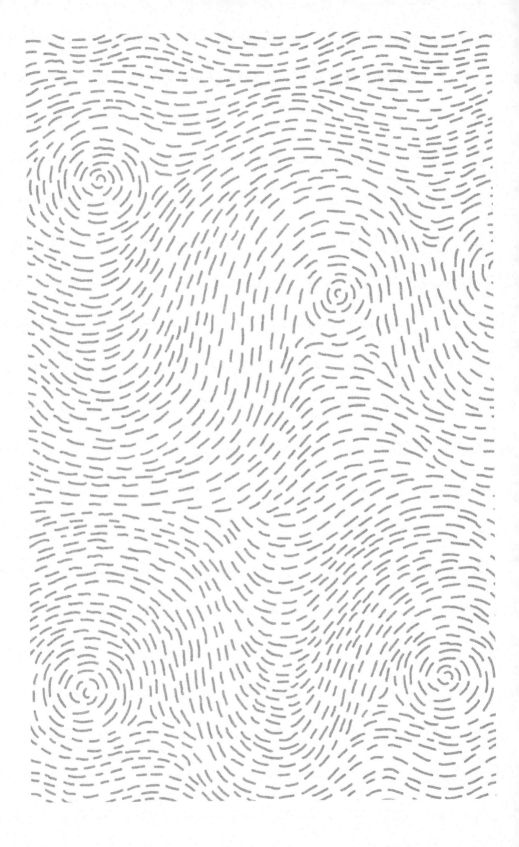

Basic Snacks

Here is a list of snacks to incorporate into your daily routine while following the Mediterranean diet. These snacks do not require much preparation, and many can be purchased directly from the grocery store.

SNACKS UNDER 50 CALORIES:

- 1 small apple, sliced
- ½ small banana
- 1 cup blueberries
- ½ cup fruit salad
- 14 grapes
- 1 sliced kiwi fruit
- 1 small orange
- 1 peach
- 1 cup chopped watermelon
- ⅛ ounce sliced avocado
- 1 cup sliced celery
- 1 sliced tomato with 1 tablespoon grated Parmesan cheese
- 1 dark chocolate square
- 3 cups air-popped popcorn
- 4 whole-grain crackers
- 1 tablespoon hummus with celery
- ½ cup plain nonfat Greek yogurt mixed with 1 teaspoon honey
- 8 pitted kalamata olives
- ½ ounce dried turkey jerky

SNACKS UNDER 100 CALORIES:

- 1 sliced apple with 2 teaspoons peanut butter
- 1 small baked apple with cinnamon
- 1 cup unsweetened applesauce
- 1 small banana
- 3 peeled clementines
- 3 tablespoons dried fruit
- 1 cup chopped pineapple
- 3 large carrots, peeled and sliced
- 1 cup tomato soup
- 3 dark chocolate squares
- 6 cups microwave popcorn
- 15 whole almonds
- 30 shelled pistachios
- ¼ cup whole-grain granola
- 2 tablespoons toasted chickpeas

- 2 tablespoons hummus with 8 baby carrots
- 1 scoop nonfat frozen yogurt
- 2 tablespoons toasted pumpkin seeds
- 1 hard-boiled egg

Healthful Substitutions

When following a new diet, it can take time to get used to new restrictions. The great thing about the Mediterranean diet is that it isn't focused on a prescribed calorie count, and the list of restrictions isn't a mile long. In order to succeed in your new diet, focus not on what you can't have but on what healthful alternatives you can enjoy. Here is a list of healthful substitutions for unhealthful foods that you can feel free to enjoy on the Mediterranean diet.

- Substitute Greek yogurt for mayonnaise or sour cream to cut down on the fat and calories.
- Use unsweetened applesauce in place of oil and butter in your recipes for baked goods—they will turn out moist and delicious.
- If you don't have any applesauce on hand, substitute an equal amount of mashed banana or avocado.
- Rather than eating bread with your meal and croutons on your salad, try substituting a tablespoon or two of nuts as a salad-topper.
- Use unbleached flour rather than all-purpose flour in your recipes. Unbleached flour does not go through chemical bleaching processes.
- Rather than using skim milk in place of cream in thick soups, and as a result sacrificing texture, try substituting puréed potato instead.
- Swap out your reduced-fat peanut butter for all-natural peanut butter. It doesn't contain all the artificial additives and still contains healthful fats.
- In several recipes you will see pitted dates as a key ingredient. Dates are a great substitute for sugar because they are naturally sweet.
- Avoid using butter in your recipes, especially when browning meats and sautéing vegetables. Use olive oil instead.
- If you are watching your cholesterol, substitute two egg whites for one whole egg in a recipe.
- Throw away your iceberg lettuce and opt for nutrient-rich greens such as kale, spinach, and romaine lettuce.

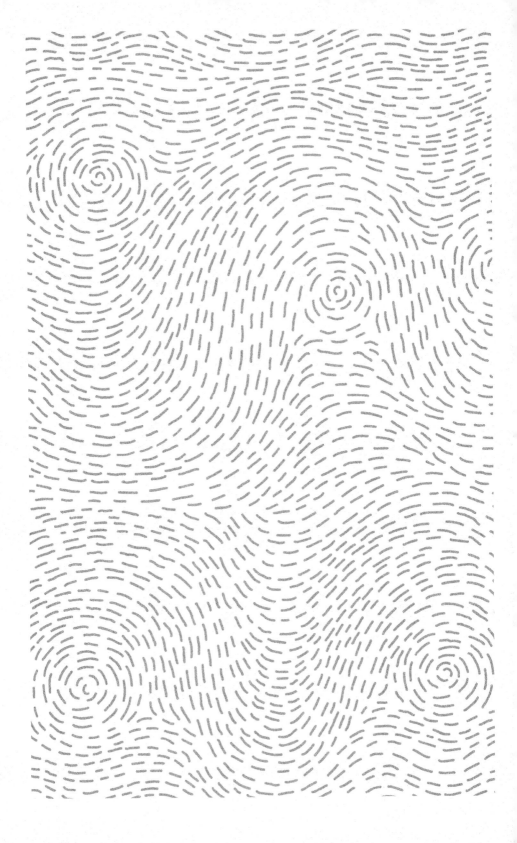

References

American Heart Association. "Mediterranean Diet." Last modified October 26, 2012. www.heart.org/HEARTORG/GettingHealthy/NutritionCenter/ Mediterranean-Diet_UCM_306004_Article.jsp.

Amidor, Toby. "Mediterranean Diet 101." Food Network. Accessed October 30, 2013. www.foodnetwork.com/healthy-eating/mediterranean-diet-101/ index.html.

Cleveland Clinic Online. "Ask the Dietician: Mediterranean Diet." Cleveland Clinic. October 2001. http://my.clevelandclinic.org/heart/prevention /askdietician/ask10_01.aspx.

Cottet, Vanessa, Mathilde Touvier, Agnès Fournier, Marina S. Touillaud, Lionel Lafay, Françoise Clavel-Chapelon, and Marie-Christine Boutron-Ruault. "Postmenopausal Breast Cancer Risk and Dietary Patterns in the E3N-EPIC Prospective Cohort Study." *American Journal of Epidemiology* 170, no. 10 (2009): 1,257–67. doi: 10.1093/aje/kwp257.

DoctorOz.com. "Dr. Oz's Mediterranean Diet Shopping List." Accessed October 30, 2013. www.doctoroz.com/videos/mediterranean-diet-shopping -list.

Goulet, Julie, Benoît Lamarche, and Simone Lemieux. "A Nutritional Inter-vention Promoting a Mediterranean Food Pattern Does Not Affect Total Daily Dietary Cost in North American Women in Free-Living Conditions." *Journal of Nutrition* 138 (January 2008): 54–9. www.ncbi.nlm.nih.gov/pubmed /18156404.

Keys, Ancel. "Epidemiological Studies Related to Coronary Heart Disease: Characteristics of Men Aged 40–59 in Seven Countries." *Acta Medica Scandinavica* 180 (1966): 4–5. doi: 10.1111/j.0954-6820.1966.tb04737.x.

Kovacs, Betty. "Mediterranean Diet." MedicineNet.com. Accessed October 30, 2013. http://www.medicinenet.com/mediterranean_diet/article.htm.

La Vecchia, Carlo. "Association between Mediterranean Dietary Patterns and Cancer Risk." *Nutrition Reviews* 67 (May 2009): 126–29. Onlinelibrary.wiley.com /doi/10.1111/j.1753-4887.2009.00174.x/full.

Lopatto, Elizabeth. "Fat and Cholesterol Aren't Only Heart Dangers of Red Meat." *Washington Post.* April 7, 2013. Articles.washingtonpost.com/2013 -04-07/national/38353911_1_gut-bacteria-carnitine-red-meat.

Mayo Clinic Staff. "Mediterranean Diet: A Heart-Healthy Eating Plan." Mayo Clinic. Accessed October 30, 2013. www.mayoclinic.com/health /mediterranean-diet/CL00011.

Mayo Clinic Staff. "Menu Planning: Eat Healthier and Spend Less." Mayo Clinic. October 25, 2011. http://www.mayoclinic.com/health/menu -planning/MY00753.

Oldways Preservation Trust. "Mediterranean Diet 101." Accessed October 30, 2013. Oldwayspt.org/resources/heritage-pyramids/get-started-go-med.

Oldways Preservation Trust. "Mediterranean Diet and Health." Accessed October 30, 2013. Oldwayspt.org/resources/heritage-pyramids/mediterranean -diet-pyramid/med-diet-health.

Oldways Preservation Trust. "Tips for Women." Accessed October 30, 2013. http://oldwayspt.org/resources/heritage-pyramids/mediterranean-diet -pyramid/tips-women.

Romaguera, Dora, Teresa Norat, Traci Mouw, Anne M. May, Christina Bamia, Nadia Slimani, Noemie Travier, et al. "Adherence to the Mediterranean Diet Is Associated with Lower Abdominal Adiposity in European Men and Women." *Journal of Nutrition* 139, no. 9 (July 2009): 1,728–37. doi:10.3945 /jn.109.108902.

Science Daily. "New Year's Resolution No. 1: Prevent Cancer, Use Olive Oil." Accessed November 25, 2013. http://www.sciencedaily.com/releases/2006/12 /061211221122.htm.

Sofi, Francesco, Francesca Cesari, Rosanna Abbate, Gian Franco Gensini, and Alessandro Casini. "Adherence to Mediterranean Diet and Health Status: Meta-Analysis." *British Medical Journal* 337 (September 2008): a1,344–50. www.bmj.com/content/337/bmj.a1344.

U.S. News & World Report. "Mediterranean Diet." Last modified September 23, 2013. Health.usnews.com/best-diet/mediterranean-diet.

Index

CPSIA information can be obtained at www.ICGtesting.com
Printed in the USA
BVOW06s0731280716

PP7224400001B/3/P